OXFORD MEDICAL PUBLI

ICHPPC-2-Defined

ICHPPC-2-Defined

(International Classification of Health Problems in Primary Care)

Third edition

ICHPPC-2 is an adaptation of the *International Classification of Diseases* (*9th revision*) intended for use in General Medicine (*ICD-9-GM*)

Prepared by the Classification Committee of WONCA (World Organization of National Colleges, Academies, and Academic Associations of General Practitioners/Family Physicians)

Oxford   New York   Toronto
OXFORD UNIVERSITY PRESS

Oxford University Press, Walton Street, Oxford OX2 6DP
Oxford New York Toronto
Delhi Bombay Calcutta Madras Karachi
Petaling Jaya Singapore Hong Kong Tokyo
Nairobi Dar es Salaam Cape Town
Melbourne Auckland
and associated companies in
Beirut Berlin Ibadan Nicosia

Oxford is a trade mark of Oxford University Press

First published 1983
Reprinted 1984, 1985, 1986 (twice)

British Library Cataloguing in Publication Data
World Organization of National Colleges, Academies
and Academic Associations of General Practitioners/
Family Physicians. Classification Committee
ICHPPC—2—defined.—3rd ed—(Oxford medical
publications)
1. Nosology
I. Title
616'.0012   RB115
ISBN 0–19–261426–6

Library of Congress Cataloging in Publication Data
Main entry under title:
International classification of health problems in
primary care.
(Oxford medical publications)
At head of title: ICHPPC–2 defined.
"ICHPPC–2 is an adaptation of the International
classification of diseases (9th revision) . . ."
Includes Index.
1. Nosology. I. World Organization of National
Colleges, Academies, and Academic Associations of
General Practitioners/Family Physicians. Classification
Committee. II. Series. [DNLM: 1. Classification.
2. Primary health care. WB 15 W93li]
RB115.1493 1983   616'.0012   83–2284
ISBN 0–19–261426–6

Printed in Hong Kong

Contents

Acknowledgement

This publication was supported in part by NIH Grant LM03289 from the National Library of Medicine and the Rockefeller Foundation Grant GAHS8037.

Introduction 1

The International Classification of Health Problems in Primary Care (*ICHPPC-2*) is one of the major direct and visible contributions WONCA (World Organization of National Colleges, Academies, and Academic Associations of General Practitioners/Family Physicians) has offered to the international health care community.

Another bench-mark is that *ICHPPC-2*, published in 1979, is endorsed by the World Health Organization, because of its almost complete correspondence with *ICD-9* (International Classification of Diseases, Ninth Revision).

Since the publication of *ICHPPC-2* the international forum of general practice/family practice has seen several new developments, some of which are reflected in the content of this new book. I greatly appreciate this opportunity to focus the attention on three aspects of the book which are eminently relevant for international family practice. (1) Most rubrics of *ICHPPC-2* are now defined by the members of the Classification Committee. It is a remarkable feat, notwithstanding the large cultural differences and the equally impressive language barriers characterizing an international organization like WONCA, that not only consensus has been gained by the members of the Classification Committee but in addition the book provides a homogeneous professional frame of reference, worthy of any mature scientific organization. (2) The new title is *ICD-9-General Medicine/ICHPPC-2-Defined*. The working relations between WONCA and WHO symbolize the fact that both international organizations share important goals in regard to the form and the content of primary health care. This is especially true in the field of classifications to be used by health care providers, where the ties between both organizations are strong. The newly developed 'Reason for Encounter Classification' clearly forms a joint venture between WHO and WONCA. In the field of mental health WONCA is involved in the development by WHO of a three-axial classification system enabling providers to classify psychological, social, and organic health problems. (3) The international glossary for primary care is essential not only to the collection of reliable data describing the process of primary care but also to enhancing communication on an international level between members of the 27 different national organizations which together now form WONCA.

The members of the Classification Committee deserve our gratitude for the publication of this new book and are to be applauded for their dedication which appears to be growing with time.

Arthur Hofmans, M.D.
President, the World Organization of National Colleges, Academies, and Academic Associations of General Practice/Family Medicine

Introduction 2

The unwritten social contract between the health professions and the societies they serve accord clinicians the power to 'label' the diverse manifestations of ill health encountered. This awesome power to label the problems, symptoms, complaints, conditions, and even the questions which worried individuals and their surrogates bring to formal sources of medical counsel, care, and cure has enormous implications.

Not only do the labels provide code words for discourses among health personnel but they are frequently fraught with important consequences for both patients and their families. From a policy viewpoint aggregated data based on counts of the assigned labels provide the bases for manpower training and deployment, for resource allocation and in many jurisdictions individual level data determines the payment of hospitals, physicians, and other personnel.

For all these reasons it is essential that a full range of appropriate and clearly defined labels be available for practitioners to employ at appropriate stages in the natural history of disease and ill health. Previous versions of the present Classification have evolved over the past quarter century. It was in 1958 that members of the (now Royal) College of General Practitioners in the United Kingdom first demonstrated that almost half the problems brought to family physicians could not be assigned a 'diagnosis', at least during the initial encounter with the patient, that was compatible with the available rubrics of the *International Classification of Diseases, Injuries and Causes of Death* (*ICD*). Through the initiatives of members of that College, and then of other groups of family physicians and general practitioners around the world, and more recently of the Classification Committees of the North American Primary Care Research Group (NAPCRG) and the World Organization of National Colleges, Academies and Academic Association of General Practitioners/Family Physicians (WONCA), this extension with definitions and inclusion criteria of the *International Classification of Health Problems in Primary Care* (*ICHPPC-2*) has emerged. Two major changes have occurred. First, most of the terms in the classification have been defined. To some extent this means that the present version has some of the characteristics of both a nomenclature and a classification and hence increases its utility for purposes of comparability over time and place. The availability of a defined classification does little to improve the accuracy, validity, or reliability of the diagnostic process *per se* but it does tend to increase the probability that clinicians and others who use the labels they assign will be using similar, if not identical, terms for what they perceive to be similar phenomena. Since primary medical care constitutes the great bulk (i.e. 90 per cent or more) of the care provided in any jurisdiction, the availability of this widely field-tested and critically appraised revision must be regarded as a major contribution to the provision of more rational and compassionate health services everywhere.

The second change is that the name of the classification has been altered slightly. The first version of this classification was known as *ICHPPC* and the second as *ICHPPC-2* with a notation that it was 'an adaptation of the *International Classification of Diseases* (*9th Revision*) intended for use in *General Medicine* (*ICD-9-GM*)'. The present version is now introduced as *ICHPPC-2-Defined* with the notation that it may also be referred to as *ICD-9-GM-Defined.*

This sequence of hieroglyphics could be confusing were it not for the fundamental contribution that it is hoped *ICHPPC-2-Defined* will make to the creation of a *Reason for Encounter* (*RFE*) classification that embodies a new paradigm for applying labels to the several stages at which the labelling process occurs. This new *Reason for Encounter* classification is being developed by a World Health Organization Task Force and it is seen as a major potential contribution to the Tenth Revision of what is currently the *ICD*. Many groups around the world hope that the next revision of the latter will consist of a family of classifications, or a series of classification modules, of which the primary care modules embodied in the *RFE* and *ICD-9-GM* classifications will be central features. The entire family of classifications starting with a classification of lay terms for ill health, extending through terms used in general or primary medicine to those used in hospital medicine, in the sub-specialties, and for impairments, disabilities, and handicaps, to classifications for causes of death, and for procedures could then be known as the *International Classification of Health Problems* (*Tenth Revision*).

The present classification should be regarded as a powerful, even fundamental component of this new paradigm. It is an essential instrument for appropriately labelling the panoply of problems that beset all those who seek relief from primary health care personnel for diverse manifestations of ill health. The members of the Committee responsible for this volume, and especially the Chairman, Professor Jack Froom, M.D. and Henk Lamberts, M.D., are indeed to be congratulated on completing this landmark volume.

Kerr L. White, M.D.
The Rockefeller Foundation

Introduction

After several years of successful and ever-increasing use of ICHPPC (International Classification of Health Problems in Primary Care), a new edition of this Classification has now been prepared.

The *ICHPPC-1* was derived from the *International Classification of Diseases, Eighth Revision* (*ICD-8*), which was subsequently revised as *ICHPPC-2*, in order to make it compatible with the then new revision of *ICD-9*. This new publication, as its predecessor, represents an adaptation for general practice and in addition to diagnoses, consists mainly of rubrics related to other problems encountered in primary health care. The new major feature is the fact that an attempt has been made to define by selection criteria the majority of terms used in the Classification and therefore *ICHPPC-2* becomes *ICHPPC-2-Defined*. It is expected that this modification will remarkably increase its usefulness by introducing the standardized inclusion criteria and terms in addition to the Classification.

It has to be understood that these criteria and terms are not necessarily the same as those used or being developed by the World Health Organization. This remark also applies to the International glossary for general practice/family practice (Appendix 2, p. 157). However, the World Health Organization welcomes this important effort to enhance communication with and among general practitioners and family physicians.

There is no difference between the numbering system and content of rubrics as compared to *ICHPPC-2*.

The primary health care goal of the World Health Organization (WHO) as stated at the 1978 conference on Primary Health Care in Alma Ata, USSR, is to achieve Health for all by the year 2000. It is essential that new information, appropriate to primary health care management, be collected in order to reassess the priorities and allow the planning and evaluation of the services. Such information is provided by the scheme outlined in the Classification of Primary Health Care which has so far not been adequately covered by the past decades' publications.

Karel Kupka, M.D.
Chief Medical Officer, Development of Epidemiological and Health Statistical Services, World Health Organization

Explanatory background

PURPOSE

The spectrum of ICHPPC includes the content of primary care: the health problems in people who feel ill, as well as those who consider themselves to be healthy but seek expert primary medical care evaluations and advice. ICHPPC is so devised that valid and reliable statistical comparisons may be made between morbidity or workload reports from front-line medical practices anywhere in the world.

The following features of ICHPPC bore heavily on its design, its development, and the organization for its maintenance:

a. ICHPPC represents a consensus on the content of primary care derived from the wide practical experience of many different general practitioners/family physicians from several countries.

b. Its broad-based input facilitates its adaptation to changes in concepts of health and disease, and to new developments in primary health care delivery.

c. The 'optional hierarchy' principle enables ICHPPC to accommodate recording problems of local importance and those of special interest to recorders, without threatening comparability.

d. The full spectrum of first-contact medicine is covered: ICHPPC can be used comfortably by health workers of various disciplines, in any setting from single-handed rural practice to the emergency department of a university hospital.

e. The brevity and simplicity of the list makes its use as effective for a secretary with pencil and paper as for a well-staffed medical records department with computer facilities.

f. While specifically directed towards the needs of primary care, *ICHPPC-2*, by virtue of its close alignment with the *International Classification of Diseases—Ninth Revision (ICD–9)*,[1] permits comparisons with work from other fields of medicine.

HISTORY

The classification needs of primary care first became apparent in the early 1950s as general practitioners began to record and study the content of their daily work. Standard usage became a subject of major concern as multi-practice studies were initiated and development of the *Diagnostic Index* (*E-Book*)[2,3] made every general practitioner into a potential recorder.

The first widely used classification for general practice was that of the British College of General Practitioners in 1959.[4] It underwent three revisions and was used in many countries.

Shortly thereafter, general practitioners/family physicians in other parts of the world were discovering the need for a special classification of the health problems encountered in primary care.[5-13] They derived the important underlying principles in the taxonomy of family medicine/general practice; and constructed classifications which were circulated to practitioners (usually in mimeographed format), and which were generally well received.

Many of these FP/GP taxonomers met in October 1972 at the Fifth World Conference on General Practice/Family Medicine in Melbourne, Australia. They agreed that there was a pressing need for a single classification which could be accepted and understood by family physicians/general practitioners everywhere. This goal seemed to be attainable, because roughly a third of all the rubrics in the several classifications in use at that time were common to all systems and most participants had similar concepts about the underlying principles which would have to be followed.

Before this meeting had ended, the World Organization of National Colleges, Academies, and Academic Associations of General Practitioners/Family Physicians (WONCA) established a working party with the charge to develop a tabular list based on the *International Classification of Diseases, 8th Revision*.

The working party, later to become the WONCA Classification Committee, agreed upon a list, and field-tested it in over 300 practices in nine countries, for a total of more than 100000 doctor–patient contacts. The rubric-by-rubric utilization figures and comments and suggestions from participants in the trial, formed the basis on which the trial version was modified to form *ICHPPC-1*.[14-16] On 7 November 1974, during the Sixth World Conference in Mexico City, that classification was unanimously accepted by the General Assembly of WONCA.

The first version of ICHPPC was published in 1975.[14] Within a short time WHO produced the ninth revision of the *International Classification of Diseases* (*ICD-9*), and *ICHPPC-1* was subsequently revised to *ICHPPC-2* in order to maintain comparability with the new revision of ICD. No other changes in philosophy or content were made in this version published in 1979.[19] The rubrics in the present version are unchanged from *ICHPPC-2*, except for the correction of errors, clarification of ambiguities, and addition of the inclusion criteria.

RELATIONSHIP OF *ICHPPC-2* TO *ICD-9*

The ninth revision of ICD[1] was intended to improve its usefulness for morbidity recording, and as with the 7th and 8th revisions it moved further away from its historic orientation towards the causes of death. The ninth revision to a marked degree addressed the needs of ambulatory medicine. Perhaps in response to family physicians input at several levels *ICHPPC-1* impacted on the expansion of *ICD-9*, especially so in Section XVI (Symptoms, Signs, and Ill-Defined Conditions) and Section XVIII (Supplementary Classification) with its attention to social, marital, and family problems.

The result of these changes in ICD is that, although perfect conversion is not possible, *ICHPPC-2* is much more closely aligned to *ICD-9*, than was *ICHPPC-1* to *ICD-8*. In particular, the number of ICHPPC rubrics that have a one-to-one relationship with a single ICD rubric (either at the third- or fourth-digit level of specificity) increased from 145 to 160 (39 to 44 per cent). More important, the number of ICHPPC rubrics which consist (in whole or in part) of a split ICD rubric (at its most specific level) has declined from 114 to 27 (31 to 7 per cent). For a little under half of the *ICHPPC-2* rubrics (48 per cent) comparability to *ICD-9* can be achieved by grouping together two or more rubrics of *ICD-9* (at the third- or fourth-digit level).

PLANS FOR THE FUTURE

Revisions

ICHPPC will be reviewed regularly, and will be revised at least as often as ICD. Users are encouraged to contact WONCA Classification Committee representatives from their respective countries about any difficulties encountered or suggestions to modify the classification or its definitions. Each communication will be carefully considered by the Committee.

Translations

ICHPPC-2 has been made available in languages other than English, as was the case with *ICHPPC-1*.

Clearinghouse

The Classification Committee is interested in receiving reports from ICHPPC users, including comments, questions, suggestions, and criticisms. Please write to the representative of the WONCA Classification Committee from your region, or to the Chairman of the Classification Committee, WONCA Secretariat, 70 Jolimont Rd., Jolimont, Victoria 3002, Australia.

MEMBERS OF THE WONCA CLASSIFICATION COMMITTEE

Dennis Aloysius, Bent Guttorm Bentsen, Charles Bridges-Webb, Paul Chan, Boz Fehler, Jack Froom, Klaus-Dieter Haehn, Erik Hagman, Bert Herries-Young, Pille Krogh-Jensen, Henk Lamberts, Chris Lund, David Metcalfe, Bill Patterson, Kumar Rajakumar, Philip Sive, Bob Westbury.

ACKNOWLEDGEMENT

This publication was supported in part by NIH Grant LM03289 from the National Library of Medicine and the Rockefeller Foundation Grant GAHS8037.

REFERENCES

1. *International classification of diseases: manual of the international statistical classification of diseases, injuries and causes of death,* 9th revision: World Health Organization, Geneva (1977).
2. EIMERL, T. S. A practical approach to the problem of keeping records for research purposes in general practice. *J. R. Coll. Gen. Pract.* **3,** 246–52 (1960).
3. Research Unit of the Royal College of General Practitioners: the diagnostic index. *J. R. Coll. Gen. Pract.* **21,** 609–12 (1971).
4. Research Committee of the College of General Practitioners. 'A classification of disease'. *J. R. Coll. Gen. Pract.* **2,** 140–59 (1959).
5. WESTBURY, R. C. and TARRANT, M. Classification of disease in general practice: a comparative study. *Can. Med. Assoc. J.* **101,** 82–7 (1969).
6. WESTBURY, R. C. The thorny road to an international classification of diseases in family medicine. *Fam. Physician Isr.* **4,** 214–19 (1974).
7. *Report on a National Morbidity Survey; Part 2.* National Health and Medical Research Council, Canberra (1969).
8. BRIDGES-WEBB, C. (ed.) The Australian general practice morbidity and prescribing survey 1969–1974. *Med. J. Aust. Spec. Suppl. No. 1* **2** (1976).
9. DREIBHOLZ, VON K. J. and ROHDE, P. A. Die Verdener Diagnosen-Liste. *Prakt. Arzt* **12,** 2–8 (1973).
10. FROOM, J. Classification of disease. *J. Fam. Pract.* **1,** 47–8 (1974).
11. LAMBERTS, H. De Morbiditeitsanalyse—1972 door de groepspraktijk Ommoord. *Huisarts en Wetenschap* **17,** 455–73 (1974).
12. —— idem. *Huisarts en Wetenschap* **18,** 7–39 (1975).

13. —— *idem. Huisarts en Wetenschap* **18,** 61–73 (1975).
14. *International classification of health problems in primary care.* American Hospital Association, Chicago (1975).
15. FROOM, J. The International Classification of Health Problems in Primary Care. *Med. Care* **14,** 450–4 (1976).
16. KJAR, P., MABECK, C. E., OLSEN, O. M., *et al.* Afprovning af WONCA's sygdomsklassifikation til brug i almen praksis. (The trial of the usefulness of WONCA's classification of health problems in general practice). *Ugeskr. Lug.* **139,** 1614–23 (1977).
17. BENTSEN, B. G. The accuracy of recording patient problems in family practice. *J. Med. Ed.* **5,** 311–16 (1976).
18. LAMBERTS, H. De 'International Classification of Health Problems in Primary Care' en een nieuwe patientenkaart voor de huisartsgeneeskunde. *Huisarts en Wetenschap* **18,** 165–73 (1975).
19. *ICHPPC-2 (International Classification of Health Problems in Primary Care)* (2nd edn). Oxford University Press (1979).

The definitions

Even before *ICHPPC-1* was published, it was clear to the WONCA Classification Committee that an internationally agreed list of rubrics to classify problems met in primary care would not in itself ensure the highest possible level of statistical comparability. Soon after ICHPPC was completed, therefore, the committee began to consider how to define the inclusion criteria for the use of each rubric.

This version of ICHPPC, *ICHPPC-2-Defined,* is the outcome of these deliberations. While it marks an improvement in the taxonomy of family medicine, it is not yet our ideal. Even if these inclusion criteria were perfect, there would be possibilities for intercoder variation.

THE SYSTEM OF DEFINITION

The construction of definitions can present profound difficulties and many types of definitions are possible. Attempts were made to provide THE BRIEFEST POSSIBLE DEFINITIONS WHICH WOULD REDUCE VARIABILITY IN CODING. As with the design of ICHPPC itself, inclusion criteria were chosen which make the most sense to most primary care providers. For the purpose of this publication the terms 'inclusion criteria' and, 'definition' are considered equivalent.

These considerations led to adoption of *stipulative definitions* as the general model: specifically, the use of *minimal inclusion criteria*. This needs further explanation.

For each rubric which has been defined, the reader will find one or more *criteria* which must be fulfilled to code a problem under that diagnostic title. Sometimes there is a choice of criteria; sometimes a certain number of criteria from a list must be satisfied.

Attempts were made to provide the *minimum* number of necessary criteria in order to reduce chances of miscoding. In some cases the criteria are too few to exclude all other possible conditions which might be coded mistakenly to that rubric; the aim was to exclude *most* of the conditions which might *commonly* be misclassified.

For the sake of brevity, we have only included those criteria with sufficient discriminatory value to distinguish this condition from others with which it might be confused. This is the opposite approach to textbooks, which usually list *all* the signs and symptoms found with a condition, regardless of how often each symptom or sign is found in that condition, how often it is found in other conditions or even in normal people.

Sometimes the rubric title itself adequately defines the condition. In these cases, the phrase 'As defined in the diagnostic title' is used. Even in the absence of this phrase, portions of the definition may be self-defining. To avoid errors, each rubric, its title with inclusion and exclusion criteria should be read in its entirety.

Some rubrics include more than one problem. In these cases, all or most parts of the rubric are defined separately. Parts are indicated as A, B, C, etc., with either definition or statement of lack of definition given for each part.

Attempts were not made to define every rubric, particularly residual rubrics, which contain too many disparate diagnoses for useful definition. These are labelled: 'Inclusion criteria for this rubric are not listed'. In these cases, the reader should consult the list of diagnoses included in the rubric title, or refer to the more complete list given for the relevant rubrics in *ICD-9*.

FIELD TRIAL OF THE DEFINITIONS

Draft definitions proposed by the Classification Committee were field tested in 12 countries. The field trial consisted of three parts: (1) general comments from experienced clinicians; (2) use of the inclusion criteria to code 50 consecutive encounters in practice; (3) use of the classification to code clinical vignettes, devised for the trial. Eighty-five physicians from 12 countries participated; 30 physicians from 6 countries coded encounters in their own practices, and 63 physicians from 11 countries coded the vignettes. As a result of the field test, 87 of the 282 initial definitions required modification, primarily in the direction of simplification, increased clarity, and better cross-indexing.

APPLYING THE CRITERIA AT DIFFERENT STAGES OF THE PROBLEM

The definitions are primarily designed to code the early presentation of a problem. If a problem is to be coded during a later encounter (after its modification by time or therapy) the coder should consider the historical information (e.g. normal blood pressure in a hypertensive person receiving therapy). Sometimes the condition will not change with time or treatment, and coders need only consider the criteria present at the current encounter. It is important when reporting results of a survey using the defined rubrics to note the methods used.

DISADVANTAGES OF THE SYSTEM

Clearly, this system of inclusion criteria is not without hazard. In order to improve the accuracy and reliability of statistics from primary care medicine, hard edges have been put to diagnostic concepts, many of which seem, in reality, to have blurred borders. Although sharp borders may not be needed for therapy or management, accurate data are useful for purposes of research. The use of hard-edged definitions may increase the content of residual rubrics. For coding problems which do not fully meet the given criteria, alternatives are suggested following 'Consider:'. These suggestions are in addition to those items which are excluded in the title of the rubric.

SOME POSSIBLE MISCONCEPTIONS

It is important that readers clearly understand several things which these definitions are *NOT intended to do.*

1. *They do not serve as a guide to diagnosis.* The primary purpose of the classification is to reduce chances of miscoding *after* a diagnosis has been made, and not to eliminate the possibility of diagnostic error. Minimal criteria for the inclusion of a problem in a certain rubric are listed for use after the diagnosis has already been made. The assumption is that the user will have considered the differential diagnosis for each problem, and have determined a provisional diagnosis prior to the time of coding. In most cases good practice of medicine requires far more information than is given in the definitions, to make accurate diagnoses.
2. *They do not set standards for care.* Although information derived from the use of *ICHPPC-2-Defined* may change medical concepts and ultimately impact on standards of care, these definitions are intended solely to improve the quality of statistical reporting.
3. *They do not act as a guide for therapy.* The criteria given in *ICHPPC-2-Defined* for inclusion or exclusion of a condition do not necessarily relate to the criteria for use of various therapies. For example, the practitioner may well decide that therapy for sinusitis is indicated in a patient whose findings were insufficient to fulfil the criteria listed under that diagnostic title.

SOURCES

The Committee felt no compulsion to devise new definitions; and accepted existing ones, if appropriate for the objectives given above. In fact, few existing definitions did meet those requirements because most had been prepared for research projects rather than for clinical practice and so tended to be rather cumbersome. In some cases, however, these definitions were accepted but modified to fit the needs of primary care.

If someone else's definition has been used without acknowledgement, apologies are given: imitation is the sincerest form of flattery.

Guidelines for the user

FAMILIARIZATION

Users should begin by reading the table of contents, the explanatory background, these guidelines, and the tabular classification to appreciate the overall arrangement of ICHPPC and the pattern of individual rubrics before commencing use.

OVERALL ARRANGEMENT OF ICHPPC

The eighteen sections of the classification (I to XVIII) conform to those of the *International Classification of Diseases (ICD)*. Most relate to body systems, some relate to etiology and some are neither.

Body systems:
   III   Endocrine, nutritional, and metabolic
   IV   Blood diseases
   V   Mental disorders
   VI   Nervous system and sense organs
   VII   Circulatory system
   VIII   Respiratory system
   IX   Genitourinary system (including breast)
   XII   Skin and subcutaneous tissue
   XIII   Musculoskeletal and connective tissue
Etiology:
   I   Infective and parasitic
   II   Neoplasms
   XIV   Congenital anomalies
   XVII   Injuries and adverse effects
Other:
   XI   Pregnancy, childbirth, and puerperium
   XV   Perinatal morbidity
   XVI   Signs, symptoms, and ill-defined conditions

XVIII   Supplementary (includes prevention procedures, family and social problems)

In general, etiology takes precedence over body system, so that neoplasms, congenital anomalies, and injuries are nearly always included in their respective sections. In the case of infections, if the specific agent causing the infection is known, it is usually classified in Section I, irrespective of site; if the infectious agent cannot be specified exactly, it is classified under the appropriate body system. For example, proven streptococcal tonsillitis is classified under infectious diseases (Section I), but tonsillitis is classified under the respiratory system (Section VIII). Unfortunately, there are exceptions, for example influenza, which is classified under the respiratory system.

Conditions occurring during pregnancy or the puerperium are usually classified in Section XI, 'Pregnancy, childbirth, and puerperium', if they affect or are related to pregnancy in any way. Similarly, most conditions affecting infants in the first month of life are classified in Section XV, 'Perinatal morbidity and mortality'.

Signs, symptoms, and ill-defined conditions are grouped in section XVI, but also many are included in the several body system sections. These should be used only when a more specific problem cannot be identified, since this is a classification of problems and not of reasons for encounter, nor of manifestations of disease.

The supplementary section (XVIII) contains some procedures. These should be coded only when it is not possible to link them with an underlying problem codable elsewhere, since this is a classification of problems and not of processes and procedues in primary care.

TABULAR LIST

Explanation of the columns (numbered from left to right)

Column 1

gives position numbers from 1 to 378. In *ICHPPC-1*, these ran sequentially. In *ICHPPC-2*, the numbers have not been changed for any single rubric, but some have been deleted and others are now out of numerical sequence (indicated in parentheses). For this edition all position numbers are inserted in sequence with details given for deletions or for current position.

Column 2

gives the four-digit 'ICHPPC Code'. Notice that the ICHPPC Code is left-hand justified; if one of the three-digit code numbers is written or printed, it must be followed by a character (a hyphen is used here, but any non-alphanumeric symbol will do) to move the number to the left.

Column 3

contains a description of each rubric, with *inclusion* and *exclusion* criteria. Exclusion terms are followed by a reference to the appropriate position and ICHPPC Codes.

Definitions

Most rubrics have criteria which must be met if the problem is to be coded to that rubric. These should be read in conjunction with the rubric title, together with its inclusion and exclusion terms. Sometimes there are suggested alternative rubrics for coding problems which do not meet the criteria, introduced by the word 'Consider:'.

Abbreviations and conventions

and   and, and/or
incl.   includes. This term denotes those problems which are included in the rubric.
excl.   excludes. This term denotes those problems which are *not* included in the rubric: they should be coded to the rubric shown in parentheses after each exclusion term.
NEC   Not elsewhere classified. When coding a rubric containing this phrase, consider whether the problem could be assigned to one that is more specific.
NOS   Not otherwise specified. When coding a rubric containing this phrase be certain that the diagnosis must be expressed in non-specific terms, rather than one that is more specific.
NYD   Not yet diagnosed. This is a subset of 'NOS'; the diagnosis is expressed in general terms because the diagnostic work-up is not yet complete.

Residual rubrics are found at the end of a section or subsection; their description includes the word '. . . other . . .'. Clearly 'NEC' is implied for all of the terms in these rubrics. A knowledge of the boundaries of this section or subsection is required for the best use of the classification. If in doubt, consult the alphabetical index of *ICHPPC-2-Defined* or *ICD-9* (see below).

Section XVI: Symptoms, signs, and ill-defined conditions. The phrases 'NEC', 'NOS', and 'NYD' could apply to all the rubrics in this section, although they are not usually included in the description. The rules for coding these rubrics are the same as they would be if these phrases were included.

Spelling. For the sake of brevity, the American spelling convention has been adopted; thus esophagus, edema, hemorrhoids, anemia, etc. Also, for the sake of brevity, the masculine pronoun is used throughout. For the purposes of this publication the terms 'general practice' and 'family medicine' are considered equivalent.

Punctuation has been held to a minimum for the sake of brevity and to assist machine processing.

Column 4

gives the equivalent codes in *ICD-9* (the ninth revision of the *International Classification of Diseases* published by the World Health Organization) for each rubric; 'ex.' indicates that the ICD Codes which follow are not found in this rubric (e.g. in Position Number 25, '112 (ex. 112.1, 112.2)' means that all of the ICD Code 112 except 112.1 and 112.2 is contained in this rubric).

ALPHABETICAL INDEX

The basic arrangement of the alphabetical index is by underlying condition, with sites and other modifiers listed in alphabetical order under the lead term. Conditions expressed by adjectives appear in the list following the lead term. Each entry is accompanied by the position number, the ICHPPC Code, and the page number, and sometimes by a cross-reference to another lead term. The code number given in the alphabetical list should be checked in the tabular list to be certain that the classification is correct. Remember that spelling is in the American convention: 'ae' and 'oe' are contracted to 'e'.

CONDENSED TITLES

Each rubric has been given a condensed title, consisting of 35 characters and spaces or less, designed for machine processing and computer printouts.

OPTIONAL HIERARCHY

Clearly no single international classification can fulfil every need for every user; inevitably users will sometimes want to separate certain problems contained in a single rubric. If this problem arises, either because of increased incidence of a condition in one area or because of the special interests of the recorder, it can be solved by assigning special 'in-house' code numbers to that condition. Some rubrics include definitions of parts of the whole which will assist coding if optional hierarchy is used. Provided that this rubric is put together with all its parts in its original ICHPPC rubric when tabulations are made and results published, there will be no loss of the comparability, which is the main purpose of ICHPPC.

CODING SYMBOLS

One of the unusual features of ICHPPC is that two code numbers are provided to identify each rubric; each, however, has certain advantages. The 'Position Number' consists of only three characters, a distinct advantage in cerebral and electronic data handling; it is designed to remain unchanged as ICHPPC is revised. The 'ICHPPC Code' closely approximates the ICD Code (for 44 per cent of the rubrics it is identical) which is valuable for some uses, especially where diagnostic data are required for billing.

Other coding systems have been suggested: in particular a mnemonic alphabetical system has been proposed which has great merit (it is obtainable through the WONCA Secretariat at the address given above). The user may use whatever system suits his needs best, provided that the content of each rubric is unchanged. It is the official policy of the Classification Committee that *Position Numbers* should always be used for the *publication* of results or *discussion* of ICHPPC.

WRITE-INS

Users are advised to write down terms which are used locally, but which are not to be found in the tabular or alphabetical list. A synonym or closely related term in ICHPPC should be used for assigning the appropriate rubric, and the preferred term should be entered in the tabular or alphabetical list for future reference.

GENERAL RULES FOR CODING

Among the several purposes of recording and coding health problems, three principal uses emerge. They are:
(1) to calculate the incidence and prevalence of morbid conditions within a defined population;
(2) to calculate work load in terms of health problems encountered by the health care provider;
(3) to establish a diagnostic index for retrieval of medical records of patients by separate diagnoses.

Although some methods of recording permit retrieval of data for all three purposes, others do not; and, it is therefore useful to consider the ultimate use(s) of the data prior to the establishment of the system of recording.

For studies of incidence, only first contacts for new episodes of illness should be recorded. For prevalence, recording may occur at any encounter during the episode of illness, but only one contact for that episode should be recorded. Work load studies require a record of every problem dealt with for every patient encounter.

To establish a diagnostic index for the purpose of retrieval of cohorts of patients with the same diagnosis, it is necessary to record the health problem on only one occasion. The date(s) of entry recorded in the index is less important than dates recorded for incidence or work load studies (i.e. the date must coincide with the time the problem is currently active, but need not reflect whether or not the problem began or was actively dealt with on the date of that encounter).

Users are encouraged to record the full spectrum of diagnoses in their practice, including organic, psychological, and social health problems. Formulations should be recorded at the highest level of diagnostic refinement of which the user can be confident. It is desirable to use the minimum number of rubrics which, in the opinion of the health care provider, fully describes the problem.

In general, the definitions are most useful for incidence studies. When used for other purposes, the recorder must decide to what extent historical data will be used or required. For example, at the first encounter with a new health care provider, a diabetic or hypertensive patient, already under therapy, may fail to fulfil criteria given for those diagnoses. Recorders should decide on a standard method of addressing this issue prior to instituting a system of recording or beginning a study which involves the use of these definitions.

SOME ASSUMPTIONS

It is assumed that users of *ICHPPC-2-Defined* will employ a recording system capable of documenting multiple problems for each patient encounter. For most of the purposes detailed under 'General rules for coding' parallel recording of the patient's age and sex, and status of the problem (e.g. new, recurrence, followup, modified diagnoses, previously diagnosed elsewhere) are useful adjuncts, but for some studies a more complete demographic data base for each patient will be required.

CODING OBSCURE PROBLEMS

If the problems cannot be located readily in the tabular list, the following procedure is advised:

a. Consult the alphabetical list of *ICHPPC-2-Defined* using the lead term (main entry) which is usually the name of the disease or health problem, rather than its anatomic location. For example:

Cyst
  Bartholin
or
  Eczema
    Atopic

b. For terms not present in the *ICHPPC-2-Defined* index, use the alphabetical index (Volume 2) of *ICD-9* to obtain the code number which can be matched with those in column 4 (Comparable ICD-9 Codes).

c. Assign the *ICHPPC-2-Defined* code (either column 1—Position Number or column 2—ICHPPC Code, depending upon which system is used) that matches the comparable ICD-9 Code.

TYPE OF CODER

The Classification is designed primarily for 'peripheral coding' (i.e. the health care provider not only establishes the diagnosis, but assigns the appropriate code number as well). Other systems involve 'central coding' in which the provider records the diagnosis, but code assignment is made by a secretary or records technician. If the latter method is employed, users should provide the necessary training for persons entrusted to making code assignments. It is expected, however, that use of the criteria given for definitions will be the responsibility of the health care provider.

QUICK GUIDE FOR USERS

1. To avoid errors, each rubric, its title (with inclusion and exclusion items and the definitions) should be read in its entirety.
2. Definitions contain the *minimal* number of criteria necessary to permit inclusion in the diagnostic title.
3. For those rubrics labelled 'Inclusion criteria for this rubric are not listed', consult the list of diagnoses included in the rubric or, for a more complete list, refer to the relevant rubrics in *ICD-9*.
4. Consult the definition *after* the diagnosis has been formulated. If the criteria given in the definitions cannot be fulfilled, consult other rubrics suggested by the term 'consider'.
5. The definitions are *not* intended to be used as a guide to therapeutic decisions.

6. Coding of diagnoses should occur at the highest level of specificity possible for that patient encounter. In most cases etiology (if known) is coded rather than clinical manifestations.
7. When the principal content of the encounter is a procedure, code the diagnoses linked to that procedure (e.g. 'removal of sutures'— code 'laceration', or 'injection of desensitization extract'—code 'hay fever').
8. It is best to adopt and maintain only one numbering system; either the position number or the ICHPPC number. For users who require ICD-9 numbers, suggestions are given in the following reference: Froom, J. and Schneeweiss, R. Use of the International Classification of Health Problems in Primary Care (ICHPPC-2) for reimbursement. *J. Fam. Pract.* **11,** 609–20 (1980).
9. It is useful to become thoroughly familiar with the contents of each section of the tabular list prior to beginning use of the Classification.
10. Decide for which purpose(s) data derived from this classification will be applied (e.g. incidence, prevalence, work load, diagnostic index) *prior* to beginning use of this classification (see 'general rules for coding').

THE GLOSSARY

'An International Glossary for Primary Care' is contained in Appendix 2 of this publication. Definitions of those terms most commonly used to describe the process of primary care are given. Equivalent, but different terms used in the several countries represented in WONCA are provided, when appropriate. The Glossary is intended as an adjunct to *ICHPPC-2-Defined* and should be consulted prior to reporting data derived from its use. Suggestions for modifications or criticisms of the Glossary should be addressed to members of the WONCA Classification Committee.

Abbreviation key

&	and/ and/or
( )	is out of sequence
EXCL	excluding
INCL	including
NEC	not elsewhere classified
NOS	not otherwise specified
NYD	not yet diagnosed
WO	without
W/WO	with or without

Tabular classification of health problems

Position no.	ICHPPC code	List of diseases, disorders, and health problems, with inclusion criteria	Comparable ICD-9 codes

I. INFECTIOUS AND PARASITIC DISEASES

1   **008-**   **Intestinal disease of proven infective origin**   001–008.6
incl. bacterial food poisoning; enteritis caused by a specified virus:
Inclusion in this rubric requires:
A symptomatic patient with *one* of the following:
(a) Isolation of pathogenic bacteria, virus, or protozoan form from either the stool or from food ingested by the affected person
(b) Serological evidence of bacterial or viral infection in affected person
Consider: (2, **009-**) Intestinal disease, presumed infective;
(*339*, **V01-**) Contacts, carriers of infective/parasitic disease

2   **009-**   **Intestinal disease—presumed to be infective,**   008.8, 009
of either unspecified viral or unkown origin
incl. diarrhea presumed to be infective
excl. chemical-induced gastroenteritis (*153*, **536-**), (*159*, **558-**); diarrhea, not presumed to be infective cause not yet determined, and NOS (*159*, **558-**); non-infective (specified) enteritis and gastroenteritis (*159*, **558-**); functional digestive disorders (*159*, **558-**), (*161*, **5640**), (*167*, **579-**); vomiting, not presumed to be infective, cause not yet determined, and NOS (*274*, **7870**)
As defined in the diagnostic title

3   —   (*Deleted*)

4   **011-**   **Tuberculosis, all sites**   010–018, 137
incl. late-effects; recent positive conversion of TB skin test
Inclusion in this rubric requires one *of the following:*
(a) Demonstration of Mycobacterium tuberculosis
(b) Characteristic appearance on X-ray
(c) Characteristic histological appearance
(d) Recent conversion to a positive tuberculin skin test, not following immunization

5   **5119**   (*See after position number 141*)

Position no.	ICHPPC code	List of diseases, disorders, and health problems, with inclusion criteria	Comparable ICD-9 codes
6	033-	**Whooping cough** *incl.* parapertussis and pertussis syndrome *Inclusion in this rubric requires* one *of the following:* (a) Respiratory infection with a characteristic staccato paroxysmal cough ending with a high-pitched inspiratory whoop (b) Respiratory infection with persistent cough (three weeks) in a contact with known pertussis (c) Demonstration of bordetella pertussis *Consider: (270,* **7862**) Cough, or acute respiratory infections in section VIII	033
7	034-	**Strep. throat (proven), scarlet fever, erysipelas** *Inclusion in this rubric requires:* **A.** *For strep. throat*—two *of the following:* (a) Acute inflammation of the throat (b) Demonstration of Streptococcus pyogenes (c) Rising antistreptolysin-O titer *Consider: (135,* **463-**) Tonsillitis **B.** *For scarlet fever*—both *of the following:* (a) Acute febrile illness with characteristic rash (b) Suspected or proven streptococcal infection of throat or skin *Consider: (14,* **057-**) Pyrexia with rash NOS **C.** *For erysipelas—the following:* An acute nonpruritic raised indurated inflammatory lesion of the skin, characterized by a well-defined border *Consider: (292,* **7821**) Non-specific skin eruption	034, 035
8	045-	**Poliomyelitis and other enterovirus diseases of the central nervous system** *incl.* late-effects; aseptic meningitis; slow virus infections *Inclusion criteria for this rubric are not listed*	045–048, 138
9	052-	**Chickenpox** *Inclusion in this rubric requires:* A vesicular exanthem which appears in successive crops, with the lesions evolving rapidly from superficial papules to vesicles and eventually to scabs *Consider: (14,* **057-**) Pyrexia with rash NOS	052
10	053-	**Herpes zoster** *Inclusion in this rubric requires:* A unilateral eruption over the area of one or more dermatomes; vesicular lesions evolve from papules and may progress to pustules or scabs	053

Position no.	ICHPPC code	List of diseases, disorders, and health problems, with inclusion criteria	Comparable ICD-9 codes
11	**054-**	**Herpes simplex, all sites** *Inclusion in this rubric requires* one *of the following:* (a) Small vesicles with characteristic appearance and location which evolve to painful ulcers and scabs (b) Herpetic whitlow, dendritic ulcer, and other conditions listed in *ICD-9*	054

12	**055-**	**Measles**
		incl. complications
		excl. German measles (*13*, **056-**)
		Inclusion in this rubric requires one *of the following*
		(a) Serological evidence of acute measles
		(b) *Two* of the following:
		   (i) Prodrome including injected conjunctivae, fever, and cough
		   (ii) White specks on a red base in the mucous membranes of the cheek (Koplik's spots)
		   (iii) Confluent maculopapular eruption spreading over the face and body
		(c) An atypical exanthem in a partially immune person during an epidemic of measles
		Consider: (*14*, **057-**) Pyrexia with rash NOS
			055

13	**056-**	**Rubella** *excl.* Roseola infantum (*14*, **057-**) *Inclusion in this rubric requires* one *of the following:* (a) An acute exanthem with enlarged lymph nodes, most prominently suboccipital and post-auricular, with a macular rash on the face, spreading to the trunk and proximal portions of the limbs (b) Serological evidence of rubella infection *Consider:* (*14*, **057-**) Pyrexia with rash NOS	056
14	**057-**	**Other viral exanthems** *incl.* pyrexia with rash NOS; roseola infantum *Inclusion criteria for this rubric are not listed*	057

Position no.	ICHPPC code	List of diseases, disorders, and health problems, with inclusion criteria	Comparable ICD-9 codes

15	**070-**	**Viral hepatitis**
		 incl. all hepatitis presumed viral
		 excl. hepatitis NOS (*165*, **571-**)
		 Inclusion in this rubric requires one *of the following:*
		 (a) *All* of the following:
		   (i) No evidence of other liver disease or exposure to liver toxins
		   (ii) Jaundice
		   (iii) Enlarged tender liver
		   (iv) Acute onset of illness under age 40 years
		 (b) *All* of the following:
		   (i) No evidence of other liver disease or exposure to liver toxins
		   (ii) Exposure to source of infection within appropriate incubation period
		   (iii) Elevated serum level of appropriate liver enzymes
		 (c) Serological evidence of an acute infection
		 (d) Characteristic histological appearance
			070

16	**072-**	**Mumps** *incl.* mumps orchitis *Inclusion in this rubric requires* one *of the following:* (a) Acute non-suppurative, non-erythematous diffuse tender inflammation of one or more salivary glands (b) Acute mumps infection demonstrated by culture or serology (c) Orchitis in a person exposed to mumps following appropriate incubation period *Consider:* (*149*, **528-**) Salivary calculus; (*296*, **7822**) Mass or localized swelling	072
17	**075-**	**Infectious mononucleosis, glandular fever** *Inclusion in this rubric requires* three *of the following:* (a) Pharyngotonsillitis (b) Lymphadenopathy not confined to anterior cervical nodes (c) Splenomegaly (d) Atypical lymphocytes on blood smear (e) Abnormal heterophile antibody titer or EB virus titer *Consider:* (*63*, **2891**) Chronic lymphadenitis; (*133*, **460-**) Acute upper respiratory tract infection; (*135*, **463-**) Tonsillitis; (*266*, **7856**) Enlarged lymph nodes	075

Position no.	ICHPPC code	List of diseases, disorders, and health problems, with inclusion criteria	Comparable ICD-9 codes
18	077-	**Conjunctivitis, caused by a virus or chlamydia** *incl.* viral pharyngoconjunctivitis *excl.* conjunctivitis NOS (*92*, **3720**) *Inclusion in this rubric requires:* Inflammation of the conjunctivae from which a virus or chlamydia are cultured or occurs during an epidemic of viral or chlamydial conjunctivitis *Consider:* (*92*, **3720**) Conjunctivitis NOS	077
19	0781	**Warts, all sites** *incl.* 'venereal' and plantar warts; verruca vulgaris; condylomata accuminata *excl.* seborrheic or senile (*277*, **709-**) *Inclusion in this rubric requires* one *of the following:* (a) Characteristic appearance of lesions (b) Characteristic histological appearance	078.1
20	0799	**Viral infection unspecified** *excl.* influenza (*139*, **487-**); viral exanthems (*14*, **057-**) *Inclusion in this rubric requires:* Presumed virus infection of unspecified nature or site	079.9
21	084-	**Malaria** *Inclusion in this rubric requires* one *of the following:* (a) Intermittent fever with chills and rigors in a resident of, or recent visitor to, a malarial region (b) Demonstration of malarial parasite forms in the peripheral blood *Consider:* (*291*, **7806**) Fever of undetermined cause	084
22	090-	**Syphilis, all sites and stages** *Inclusion in this rubric requires* one *of the following:* (a) Demonstration of *Treponema pallidum* on microscopy (b) Positive serological test specific for syphilis	090–097

Position no.	ICHPPC code	List of diseases, disorders, and health problems, with inclusion criteria	Comparable ICD-9 codes
23	098-	**Gonorrhea, all sites**	098

Gonorrhea, all sites
Inclusion in this rubric requires one *of the following:*
(a) Purulent urethral or vaginal discharge in a contact with a proven case
(b) Gram negative intra-cellular diplococci demonstrated in discharge
(c) Culture of *Neisseria gonorrhea*
Consider: (*372*, **0994**) Urethritis, non-specific; (*172*, **597-**) Urethritis, non-venereal; (*300*, **7889**) Urethral discharge NYD
098

(*372*) **0994** **Nonspecific urethritis** 099.4
excl. other urethritis (*172*, **597-**)
Inclusion in this rubric requires both *of the following:*
(a) Urethral discharge, presumed sexually transmitted
(b) Failure to find *Neisseria gonorrheae* by microscopy or culture
Consider: (*300*, **7889**) Urethral discharge NYD; (*172*, **597-**) Urethritis, non-venereal

24 **110-** **Dermatophytosis and Dermatomycosis** 110, 111
incl. athlete's foot; tinea; ringworm; onychomycosis
Inclusion in this rubric requires one *of the following:*
(a) Characteristic clinical appearance
(b) Demonstration of the fungus on microscopy or culture

25 **112-** **Monilia infection, candidiasis, any sites except urogenital** 112 (ex. 112.1, 112.2)
incl. oral cavity, thrush, rectal and anal mucosa
Inclusion in this rubric requires one *of the following:*
(a) Characteristic clinical appearance
(b) Demonstration of candida on microscopy or culture in a patient with appropriate signs or symptoms

26 **1121** **Urogenital candidiasis—proven** 112.1, 112.2
incl. monilial infection of vagina or cervix
Inclusion in this rubric requires both *of the following:*
(a) Inflamed urogenital mucosa or skin
(b) Demonstration of candida on microscopy or culture
Consider: (*179*, **605-**) Balanitis; (*185*, **6161**) Vaginitis

Position no.	ICHPPC code	List of diseases, disorders, and health problems, with inclusion criteria	Comparable ICD-9 codes
27	1310	**Urogenital trichomoniasis—proven** *excl.* leukorrhea NOS (*194*, **629-**) *Inclusion in this rubric requires* both *of the following:* (a) Inflamed urogenital mucosa (b) Demonstration of trichomonads on microscopy *Consider:* (*179*, **605-**) Balanitis; (*185*, **6161**) Vaginitis	131.0
28	127-	**Oxyuriasis, pinworms, and all other helminths** *incl.* creeping eruption; intestinal parasites NOS; trichiniasis *Inclusion in this rubric requires* one *of the following:* (a) Demonstration of helminth in adult form, larvae, or ova (b) Positive skin tests (c) Positive serology	120–129
29	132-	**Pediculosis and other skin infestations** *incl.* larvae, maggots, sandfleas, leeches *Inclusion in this rubric requires:* Demonstration of infesting organisms	132, 134
30	133-	**Scabies and other acariases** *Inclusion in this rubric requires* one *of the following:* (a) Presence of characteristic burrows on a pruritic skin (b) Demonstration of organisms by microscopy	133
31	136-	**All other infective and parasitic diseases** *incl.* brucellosis; cowpox; Coxsackie diseases; meningococal infections; molluscum contagiosum; rickettsial disease; smallpox; trachoma; venereal disease, other, NEC; Vincent's angina; viral encephalitis; (see ICD for other inclusions) *Inclusion criteria for this rubric are not listed*	020–027, 030–032, 036–041, 049–051, 060–074, 076, 078 ex. 078.1, 079 ex. 079.9, 080–083, 085–088, 099 ex. 099.4, 100–104, 114–118, 130, 131 ex. 131.0, 135, 136, 139

Position no.	ICHPPC code	List of diseases, disorders, and health problems, with inclusion criteria	Comparable ICD-9 codes

II. NEOPLASMS

In most parts of the world, the requirement for the diagnosis of malignant neoplasm includes a characteristic histological appearance, although it is recognized that in some cases the diagnosis may be made on clinical grounds alone. The Committee recommends that prior to biopsy most cases be coded to (*46*, **239-**) Neoplasms, not yet determined whether benign or malignant; or, if in doubt as to whether the cause is neoplasm (*296*, **7822**) Mass and localized swelling, or to the dominant sympton. Following biopsy and histology, coding should be to the appropriate rubric.

Malignant Neoplasms

| *32* | **151-** | **Esophagus, stomach, large bowel, rectum, anus**
 Inclusion in this rubric requires:
 Characteristic histological appearance
 Consider: (*39*, **199-**) Other malignant neoplasms
 (when primary site is uncertain); (*46*, **239-**)
 Neoplasms NYD whether benign or malignant
 (when histology is not available) | 150, 151, 153, 154 |

| *33* | **162-** | **Larynx, trachea, bronchus and lung**
 Inclusion in this rubric requires:
 Characteristic histological appearance
 Consider: (*39*, **199-**) Other malignant neoplasms
 (when primary site is uncertain); (*46*, **239-**)
 Neoplasms NYD whether benign or malignant
 (when histology is not available) | 161, 162 |

| *34* | **173-** | **Skin, subcutaneous tissue**
 incl. melanoma
 Inclusion in this rubric requires:
 Characteristic histological appearance
 Consider: (*39*, **199-**) Other malignant neoplasms
 (when primary site is uncertain); (*46*, **239-**)
 Neoplasms NYD whether benign or malignant
 (when histology is not available) | 172, 173 |

| *35* | **174** | **Breast**
 Inclusion in this rubric requires:
 Characteristic histological appearance
 Consider: (*39*, **199-**) Other malignant neoplasms
 (when primary site is uncertain); (*46*, **239-**)
 Neoplasms NYD whether benign or malignant
 (when histology is not available) | 174, 175 |

Position no.	ICHPPC code	List of diseases, disorders, and health problems, with inclusion criteria	Comparable ICD-9 codes
36	**180-**	**Female genital tract** *incl.* adnexa; cervix (*incl. in situ*); uterus; vagina; vulva *Inclusion in this rubric requires:* Characteristic histological appearance *Consider:* (*39*, **199-**) Other malignant neoplasms (when primary site is uncertain); (*46*, **239-**) Neoplasms NYD whether benign or malignant (when histology is not available); (*184*, **622-**) Cervical leukoplakia; (*376*, **7950**) Nonspecific abnormal Pap smear	179, 180, 182–184, 233.1
37	**188-**	**Urinary and male genital tract** *incl.* bladder; kidney; prostate; testis *Inclusion in this rubric requires:* Characteristic histological appearance *Consider:* (*39*, **199-**) Other malignant neoplasms (when primary site is uncertain); (*46*, **239-**) Neoplasms NYD whether benign or malignant (when histology is not available)	185–189
38	**201-**	**Hodgkin's disease, the lymphomata, the leukemias** *incl.* multiple myeloma *Inclusion in this rubric requires:* Characteristic histological appearance *Consider:* (*39*, **199-**) Other malignant neoplasms (when primary site is uncertain); (*46*, **239-**) Neoplasms NYD whether benign or malignant (when histology is not available)	200–208
39	**199-**	**Other malignant neoplasms** *incl.* secondary and metastatic neoplasms where primary site is unknown; carcinoma *in situ* (*excl.* carcinoma *in situ* of cervix (*36*–**180**)); carcinoma of pancreas *Inclusion in this rubric requires:* Characteristic histological appearance *Consider:* (*46*, **239-**) Neoplasms NYD whether benign or malignant (when histology is not available)	140–149, 152. 155–160, 163–171, 181, 190–199, 230–232, 233 ex. 233.1, 234

Position no.	ICHPPC code	List of diseases, disorders, and health problems, with inclusion criteria	Comparable ICD-9 codes

Benign Neoplasms

40	**214-**	**Lipoma, any site** *Inclusion in this rubric requires* one *of the following:* (a) Characteristic, soft, well demarcated subcutaneous tumor (b) Characteristic macroscopic or histological appearance	214
41	**216-**	**Skin** *incl.* mole; pigmented nevus *excl.* hemangioma (*44*, **228-**); residual hemorrhoidal skin tags (*130*, **455-**); seborrheic or senile warts (*227*, **709-**); hyperkeratoses (*227*, **709-**); solar keratoses (*227*, **709-**) *Inclusion in this rubric requires:* Tumor showing characteristic appearance or histology *Consider:* (*46*, **239-**) Neoplasm NYD as benign malignant; (*296*, **7822**) Mass and localized swelling	216
42	**217-**	**Breast** *excl.* simple cysts, chronic cystic disease (*181*, **610-**); skin of breast (*41*, **216-**) *Inclusion in this rubric requires:* A benign breast tumor proven histologically *Consider:* (*182*, **611-**) Lump in breast NOS	217
43	**218-**	**Fibroids and other tumors of uterus** *incl.* cervical polyp (adenomatous); myoma *excl.* mucous cervical polyp (*184*, **622-**) *Inclusion criteria are not listed for part of this rubric* *For optional hierarchy, inclusion in this rubric requires:* **A.** *For fibroid*—one *of the following:* (a) Generalized enlargement of the uterus with no evidence of pregnancy or malignancy (b) Single or multiple firm tumors of the uterus **B.** *For other tumors of the uterus:* *Inclusion criteria for this part of the rubric are not listed*	218, 219

Position no.	ICHPPC code	List of diseases, disorders, and health problems, with inclusion criteria	Comparable ICD-9 codes
44	**228-**	**Hemangioma, lymphangioma** *incl.* angiomatous birthmarks *excl.* birthmarks NOS (*252*, **758-**) *Inclusion in this rubric requires* one *of the following:* (a) Characteristic histological appearance (b) Characteristic appearance of skin lesion	228
45	**229-**	**Other benign neoplasms** *incl.* adenomatous cyst of ovary; adenomatous polyp of cervix; anus; brain; digestive system; endocrine system; large bowel; polyposis of bowel; rectum *excl.* polyp of middle ear (*107*, **388-**); polyp of larynx or nose (*147*, **519-**); mucous polyp of cervix (*184*, **622-**); physiological cyst of ovary (*194*, **629-**) *Inclusion criteria for this rubric are not listed*	210–213, 215, 220–227, 229

Unspecified neoplasms

46	**239-**	**Neoplasms, not yet determined whether benign or malignant** *incl.* polycythemia rubra vera *excl.* carcinoma-*in-situ* (*36*, **180-**), (*39*, **199-**); breast lump NOS (*182*, **611-**); atypical or abnormal Pap smear NOS (*376*, **7950**); localized swelling (*296*, **7822**); other malignant neoplasms (*39*, **199-**) *As defined in the diagnostic title*	235–239

Position no.	ICHPPC code	List of diseases, disorders, and health problems, with inclusion criteria	Comparable ICD-9 codes

III. ENDOCRINE, NUTRITIONAL AND METABOLIC DISEASES AND IMMUNITY DISORDERS

47	**240-**	**Goiter and thyroid nodule without thyrotoxicosis** *excl.* proven neoplasm of thyroid (*39,* **199-**), (*45,* **299-**), (*46,* **239-**) *Inclusion in this rubric requires:* Enlargement of the thyroid gland with no evidence of hyperthyroidism (*48,* **242-**)	240, 241
48	**242-**	**Hyperthyroidism thyrotoxicosis,** with or without goiter *Inclusion in this rubric requires* one *of the following:* (a) Laboratory evidence of excessive thyroid hormone activity (b) *Two* of the following: (i) Tremor, weight loss, and rapid pulse (over 100/min. at rest) (ii) Eye signs (exophthalmus, lid lag, or ophthalmoplegia) (iii) Thyroid nodule or goiter	242
49	**244-**	**Hypothyroidism, myxedema, cretinism** *Inclusion in this rubric requires* one *of the following:* (a) Laboratory evidence of diminished thyroid hormone activity, or excessive thyroid stimulating hormone (b) *Four* of the following: (i) Weakness, tiredness (ii) Mental changes: apathy, poor memory, slowing (iii) Voice changes: coarser, deeper slower speech (iv) Undue sensitivity to the cold (v) Constipation (vi) Coarse puffy facial features (vii) Cool, dry, sallow skin, decreased sweating (viii) Peripheral edema	243, 244

Position no.	ICHPPC code	List of diseases, disorders, and health problems, with inclusion criteria	Comparable ICD-9 codes
50	**250-**	**Diabetes mellitus**	250

50 **250-** **Diabetes mellitus**   250

excl. hyperglycemia NOS; abnormal glucose tolerance test (*51*, **7902**)

Inclusion in this rubric requires one *of the following:*

(a) Fasting plasma glucose levels of 140 mg/dl (8 mmol/1) or more on two or more occasions

(b) An oral glucose tolerance test (75 gm of glucose) which meets *all* of the following:
   (i) One value of plasma glucose at between 0 and 2 hours of 200 mg/dl (11 mmol/1) or more
   (ii) Plasma glucose at 2 hours of 200 mg/dl (11 mmol/1) or more
   (iii) The abnormal result should not be attributable to: infection, inactivity, obesity, hypercortisolism, hyperthyroidism, surgical stress, carbohydrate restriction, diabetogenic drugs

(c) The classic symptoms of diabetes, such as polyuria, polydipsia, ketonuria, and rapid weight loss, together with gross and unequivocal elevation of plasma glucose

Note: If secondary diabetes, code primary etiology

Consider: (*51*, **7902**) Hyperglycemia

51 **7902-** (See after position number 298)

52 **260-** **Vitamin deficiency, other nutritional deficiencies**   260–269
and disorders
excl. sprue, malabsorption syndrome (*167*, **579-**)
Inclusion criteria for this rubric are not listed

53 **7833** (See after position number 294)

Position no.	ICHPPC code	List of diseases, disorders, and health problems, with inclusion criteria	Comparable ICD-9 codes
54	**274-**	**Gout**	274

excl. pseudogout and crystal arthropathies (*57,* **279-**); hyperuricemia (*51,* **7902**)
Inclusion in this rubric requires both *of the following:*
(a) *One* of the following:
   (i) Severe acute inflammation of one or more joints
   (ii) Evidence of renal failure with a past history of uric acid urinary calculus
   (iii) Clinical diagnosis of tophus
(b) *One* of the following:
   (i) Raised serum uric acid
   (ii) Uric acid deposits found on renal biopsy
   (iii) Uric acid demonstrated in a tophus
   (iv) Uric acid crystals demonstrated in the aspirate from a joint
Consider: (*231,* **725-**) Arthritis NYD or NOS

| *55* | **278-** | **Obesity** | 278 |

Inclusion in this rubric requires one *of the following:*
(a) Overweight of at least 20% according to appropriate tables
(b) Excess skin-fold thickness of at least 20% according to appropriate tables
Consider: (*338,* **V70-**) normal variation; (*338,* **V70-**) 'worried well'

| *56* | **272-** | **Disorders of lipid metabolism (hyperlipidemia, abnormalities of lipoprotein levels, and raised levels of cholesterol and triglycerides)** | 272 |

incl. congenital xanthoma
As defined in the diagnostic title

| *57* | **279** | **Other endocrine, nutritional and metabolic diseases, and immunity disorders** | 245, 246, 251–259, 270, 271, 273, 275–277, 279 |

incl. amyloidosis; congenital metabolic disorders; cystic fibrosis; diabetes insipidus; disorders of fluids, electrolytes, or acid–base balance; fluid retention; hypoglycemia; hypopituitarism; thyroiditis
Inclusion criteria for this rubric are not listed

Position no.	ICHPPC code	List of diseases, disorders, and health problems, with inclusion criteria	Comparable ICD-9 codes

IV. DISEASES OF BLOOD AND BLOOD-FORMING ORGANS

58   **280-**   **Iron deficiency anemia**   280
excl. in pregnancy, childbirth and puerperium
(*202*, **648-**)
Inclusion in this rubric requires both *of the following:*
(a) Decrease in hemoglobin or hematocrit below levels appropriate for age and sex
(b) *One* of the following:
   (i) Evidence of excessive blood loss
   (ii) Microcytic hypochromic red cells by appearance or indices in the absence of thalassemia
   (iii) Decreased serum iron and increased iron-binding capacity
   (iv) Decreased serum ferritin
   (v) Reduced hemosiderin in bone marrow
   (vi) Good response to iron administration
Consider: (*61*, **285-**) Anemia NOS

59   **281-**   **Pernicious anemia and other deficiency anemias**   281
incl. folate deficient anemia
excl. in pregnancy, childbirth and puerperium
(*202*, **648-**)
Inclusion criteria are not listed for part of this rubric
For optional hierarchy, inclusion in this rubric requires:
A. *For pernicious anemia or folic acid deficiency*—both *of the following:*
(a) Macrocytic anemia by smear or indices
(b) Decreased Vitamin B_{12} level, folate level, or positive Schilling test
B. *For other deficiency anemias:*
Inclusion criteria for this part of the rubric are not listed

Position no.	ICHPPC code	List of diseases, disorders, and health problems, with inclusion criteria	Comparable ICD-9 codes
60	282-	**Hereditary hemolytic anemias** *incl.* sickle-cell anemia; sickle-cell trait; spherocytosis; thalassemia *Inclusion criteria are not listed for part of this rubric* *For optional heirarchy, inclusion in this rubric requires:* **A.** *For sickle-cell anemia, sickle-cell trait, and thalassemia:* Characteristic findings by hemoglobin electrophoresis or smear **B.** *For spherocytosis:* Demonstration of increased osmotic fragility of red cells **C.** *For other hereditary hemolytic anemias:* *Inclusion criteria for this part of the rubric are not listed*	282
61	285-	**Other anemias** *incl.* anemia NOS *excl.* in pregnancy, childbirth and puerperium (*202,* **648-**) *Inclusion criteria for this rubric are not listed*	283–285
62	287-	**Purpura, hemorrhagic conditions, coagulation defects, abnormality of platelets** *Inclusion criteria for this rubric are not listed*	286, 287
63	2891	**Chronic and nonspecific lymphadenitis** *incl.* mesenteric lymphadenitis, acute or chronic *excl.* acute lymphadenitis, apart from mesenteric (*209,* **683-**); enlarged lymph node, not infected (*266,* **7856**) *Inclusion in this rubric requires:* **A.** *For mesenteric lymphadenitis, acute or chronic:* Demonstration of enlarged inflamed mesenteric lymph nodes by surgery, sonography, or lymphography **B.** *For other chronic and non-specific lymphadenitis:* Enlarged tender lymph nodes present for more than 6 weeks	289.1–289.3
64	288-	**Abnormal white cells** *incl.* agranulocytosis; eosinophilia; leukocytosis; lymphocytosis *excl.* leukemia (*38,* **201-**) *Inclusion in this rubric requires:* Demonstration of either abnormal quantity, morphology, or function of white blood cells	288

Position no.	ICHPPC code	List of diseases, disorders, and health problems, with inclusion criteria	Comparable ICD-9 codes
65	**2899**	**Other disorders of blood and blood-forming organs** *incl.* secondary polycythemia *excl.* primary polycythemia (*46*, **239-**) *Inclusion criteria for this rubric are not listed*	289.0, 289.4–289.9

Position no.	ICHPPC code	List of diseases, disorders, and health problems, with inclusion criteria	Comparable ICD-9 codes

V. MENTAL DISORDERS

Psychoses (except alcohol and drug induced)*

66   **294-**   Organic psychosis   290, 293, 294
incl. non-alcoholic acute or chronic delirium;
senile and presenile dementia
Inclusion in this rubric requires:
A. *For dementia not attributable to alcohol or drugs—the following:*
Chronic deterioration of intellectual functioning, with *three* of the following:
(a) Lack of orientation to time, place, or person
(b) Reduced short-term memory
(c) Reduced comprehension for abstract ideas
(d) Reduced ability to perform simple calculations
(e) Change in affect or personality
B. *For delirium or confusional state (not attributable to alcohol or drugs):*
Acute loss of intellectual functioning, accompanied by a loss of contact with reality, showing *both* of the following:
(a) *Two* of the features of dementia ((a) through (e), above)
(b) *Two* of the following:
     (i) Altered consciousness and level of attention (may fluctuate from intense preoccupation to disinterest)
     (ii) Confusion
     (iii) Delusions
     (iv) Illusions
     (v) Hallucinations
Consider: (*69,* **298-**) Psychosis, NOS

---

* Mental disorders in which impairment of mental function has developed to a degree that interferes grossly with insight, ability to meet some ordinary demands of life, or to maintain adequate contact with reality. It is not an exact or well defined term. Mental retardation is excluded. (Glossary for Chapter V of ICD-9)

Position no.	ICHPPC code	List of diseases, disorders, and health problems, with inclusion criteria	Comparable ICD-9 codes
67	**295-**	**Schizophrenia, all types**	295, 297, 298.3, 298.4

Schizophrenia, all types
incl. paranoid states and reactions
Inclusion in this rubric requires:
A disorder of at least six months' duration, which grossly impairs the patient's capacity to meet the ordinary demands of life, without evidence of primary mood disorder, primary drug abuse, or organic brain syndrome, which shows *one* of the following:
(a) Disordered thought (illusions, delusions, hallucination, or paranoid state)
(b) Disordered mood (ambivalence, constriction, or inappropriate mood)
(c) Disordered behavior (withdrawal, regression, bizarre behavior, catatonia)
Consider: (*69*, **298-**) Psychosis, NOS

68 **296-** **The affective psychoses**   296, 298.0
incl. hypomania; involutional melancholia; mania; manic-depression; psychotic depression; reactive depressive psychosis
Inclusion in this rubric requires all *of the following:*
(a) Disorder predominantly in the area of mood, showing either severe depression or marked elation and expansiveness, or the two alternating, distinguishable from the usual range of emotion
(b) Of such a degree that it grossly impedes the ability of the patient to meet the ordinary demands of life
(c) If unipolar, requires disorder of thought (delusions, hallucinations, or paranoid state)
(d) Not due to alcohol or drugs
Consider: (*69*, **298-**) Psychoses NOS; (*72*, **3004**) Depression NOS

69 **298-** **Other and unspecified psychoses**   298.2, 298.8, 298.9,
excl. alcoholic (**3031**)   299
Inclusion criteria for this rubric are not listed

Position no.	ICHPPC code	List of diseases, disorders, and health problems, with inclusion criteria	Comparable ICD-9 codes

Neuroses*

70	**3000**	**Anxiety disorder, anxiety state**	300.0

excl. Anxiety causing a somatic complaint (*71*,
3001); Anxiety depression (*72*, **3004**)
Inclusion in this rubric requires both *of the
following:*
(a) Generalized and persistent anxiety or
anxious mood, which cannot be associated
with, or is disproportionately large in
response to, a specific psycho-social
stressor, stimulus, or event
(b) No evidence of other psychological
disorders
Consider: (*77*, **308-**) Transient situational
disturbance, adjustment reaction; (*73*, **3009**)
Neuroses NOS; (*78*, **312-**) Behavior disorder

---

* Neurotic disorders are mental disorders without any demonstrable organic basis in which the
patient may have considerable insight and has unimpaired reality testing, in that he usually does not
confuse his morbid subjective experiences and fantasies with external reality. Behaviour may be
greatly affected although usually remaining within socially acceptable limits, but personality is not
disorganized. The principal manifestations include excessive anxiety, hysterical symptoms, phobias,
obsessional and compulsive symptoms, and depression. (Glossary for Chapter V of ICD-9).

Position no.	ICHPPC code	List of diseases, disorders, and health problems, with inclusion criteria	Comparable ICD-9 codes
71	**3001**	**Hysterical and hypochondriacal disorders**	300.1, 300.7, 306

3001 **Hysterical and hypochondriacal disorders**

incl. anxiety causing a somatic complaint; cardiac neurosis; compensation neurosis; conversion hysteria; factitious disorders; hyperventilation syndrome; hysterical state

excl. insomnia (*75*, **3074**); tension headache (*76*, **3078**); psychogenic disorders of sexual functions (*79*, **3027**); neurodermatitis (*218*, **698-**); malingering (*338*, **V70-**); psychogenic pain (*76*, **3078**)

Inclusion in this rubric requires:

A. *For anxiety causing a somatic complaint*—both *of the following:*
(a) Criteria for anxiety disorder (*70*, **3000**)
(b) Somatic complaint (except pain) not explainable by organic disorder or other mental disease

B. *For hypochondriasis:*
Excessive concern with health in general or with the integrity or functioning of some part of one's body or mind

C. *For conversion hysteria*—all *of the following:*
(a) Alteration of physical or mental functioning, not explainable by an organic disorder or other mental diseases
(b) Temporal relationship between psychological stimuli and symptoms
(c) Evidence of secondary gain

D. *For compensation neurosis:*
The prolongation of symptoms beyond the expected time of recovery, apparently related to expected benefit

E. *For factitious disorders:*
An attempt to deceive or falsify medical evidence, without evidence of secondary gain except that of assumption of the 'patient' role

Consider: (*73*, **3009**) Neurosis NOS

Position no.	ICHPPC code	List of diseases, disorders, and health problems, with inclusion criteria	Comparable ICD-9 codes
72	3004	**Depressive disorder (neurotic depression)** *incl.* depression NOS; anxiety depression *excl.* brief depressive stress reactions (*77*, **308-**) *Inclusion in this rubric requires* both of *the following:* (a) Absence of psychosis (b) *Three* of the following: (i) Sadness or melancholy out of proportion to psychosocial stress (ii) Suicidal thoughts or attempt (iii) Indecisiveness, decrease in interest in usual activities, or slow thinking (iv) Feelings of worthlessness, self-reproach, or inappropriate or excessive guilt (v) Early morning waking, hypersomnia, morning tiredness (vi) Anxiety, irritability, agitation *Consider:* (*68*, **296-**) Psychotic depression; (*73*, **3009**) Other neuroses; (*77*, **308-**) Transient situational disturbance, adjustment reaction	300.4, 311
73	3009	**Other neuroses** *incl.* neurasthenia; neurosis NOS; obsessive compulsive disorder; occupational neurosis; phobic state *Inclusion criteria for this rubric are not listed*	3002.2, 300.3, 300.5, 300.6, 300.8, 300.9

Other mental and psychological disorders

Position no.	ICHPPC code	List of diseases, disorders, and health problems, with inclusion criteria	Comparable ICD-9 codes
74	315-	**Specific learning disorders and delays in development of certain skills needed for schooling** *incl.* dyslexia *excl.* mental retardation (*85*, **317-**) *Inclusion criteria for this rubric are not listed*	315
75	3074	**Insomnia and other sleep disorders** *Inclusion in this rubric requires:* Any disturbance of sleep not directly attributable to any other problem	307.4

Position no.	ICHPPC code	List of diseases, disorders, and health problems, with inclusion criteria	Comparable ICD-9 codes
76	**3078**	**Tension headache, psychogenic backache and other pain of mental origin (psychalgia)** *excl.* headache NOS (*258*, **7840**); lumbalgia (*238*, **7242**); migraine (*90*, **346-**) *Inclusion in this rubric requires* both *of the following:* (a) Any pain related in timing or intensity to psychosocial stress (b) Pain not explainable by organic disorder or other mental disease	307.8
77	**308-**	**Transient situational disturbance, acute stress reaction, adjustment reaction** *incl.* bereavement; brief depressive reaction; grief reaction; may have additional code for cause (*356*, **V602**) to (*369*, **V629**) in Section XVIII *Inclusion in this rubric requires* both *of the following:* (a) Psychological symptoms closely related in time and content to a stressful event (b) Mild and transient (less that 6 months)	308, 309
78	**312-**	**Behavior disorder (any age), disturbance of emotions specific to childhood and adolescence** *incl.* delinquency; hyperkinetic child; kleptomania (any age) *excl.* character disorder (*84*, **301-**) *Inclusion criteria for this rubric are not listed*	312–314
79	**3027**	**Psychogenic disorder of sexual function** *incl.* frigidity; impotence; loss of libido; psychogenic dyspareunia; *excl.* dyspareunia NOS (*374*, **6250**); vaginismus NOS (*374*, **6250**); marital problems (*359*, **V611**) *Inclusion in this rubric requires* both *of the following:* (a) Any sexual disorder not explained by organic disorder or mental disease (b) The sexual disorder is not due to a disturbance of the marital relationship	302.7

Position no.	ICHPPC code	List of diseases, disorders, and health problems, with inclusion criteria	Comparable ICD-9 codes
80	**3031**	**Chronic abuse of alcohol** *incl.* alcoholic psychosis; alcoholism *excl.* non-dependent alcohol abuse (*81*, **3050**) *Inclusion in this rubric requires:* Excessive or repeated intake of alcohol for at least six months and *one* of the following: (a) Symptoms of withdrawal (b) Evidence of organic or psychological disorder due to alcohol toxicity (c) Pathological pattern of use (drinks, nonbeverage alcohol, binges) (d) Interfaces with normal function (social relationships, job performance, legal obligations) *Consider:* (*342*, **V10-**) Observation/care of high risk patient (if at risk for chronic alcoholism)	291, 303
81	**3050**	**Acute alcohol intoxication, drunk, and excessive alcohol intake NOS** *As defined in the diagnostic title*	305.0
82	**3051**	**Abuse of tobacco** *Inclusion in this rubric requires* one *of the following:* (a) Excessive use of tobacco (b) Use of any amount of tobacco when contraindicated in the presence of disease (e.g. chronic bronchitis, ischemic heart disease, or peripheral vascular disease) (c) Smoking is considered to be a problem by the patient	305.1
83	**3048**	**Other drug abuse, habituation, or addiction** *incl.* drug-induced psychosis: diazepam, cannabis, LSD, barbiturates, laxatives, glue sniffing, etc. *Inclusion criteria for this rubric are not listed*	292, 304, 305.2–305.9
84	**301-**	**Personality and character disorders** *Inclusion in this rubric requires* both *of the following:* (a) Deeply ingrained maladaptive pattern of behavior, recognizable by age 20 and present for at least 5 years (b) Patient or persons in his environment suffer considerably because of the behavior patterns *Consider:* (*86*, **316-**) Other mental and psychological disorders	301

Position no.	ICHPPC code	List of diseases, disorders, and health problems, with inclusion criteria	Comparable ICD-9 codes
85	**317-**	**Mental retardation** *Inclusion in this rubric requires:* Incomplete intellectual development with an IQ level of 70 or below *Note:* Other associated physical or mental disorders require additional codes	317–319
86	**316-**	**Other mental and psychological disorders** *incl.* anorexia nervosa; habit spasm; psychological causes of diseases classified elsewhere; psychological effects of head injuries; sexual deviation; tic *excl.* enuresis *not* clearly of psychological origin *(281,* **7883)** *Inclusion criteria for this rubric are not listed*	302 ex. 302.7, 307 ex. 307.4, ex. 307.8, 310, 316

Position no.	ICHPPC code	List of diseases, disorders, and health problems, with inclusion criteria	Comparable ICD-9 codes

VI. DISEASES OF THE NERVOUS SYSTEM

87	340-	**Multiple Sclerosis** *Inclusion in this rubric requires:* Exacerbations and remissions of multiple neurological manifestations with deficits disseminated in both time and site (any combination of neurological signs and symptoms is possible) *Consider: (91,* **355-**) Other nervous system diseases NEC; *(254,* **7803**) to *(259,* **7820**) Signs, Symptoms and Ill-Defined Conditions in Section XVI	340
88	332-	**Parkinsonism, paralysis agitans** *Inclusion in this rubric requires* all *of the following:* (a) Coarse tremor, improving with active purposeful movement (b) Muscular rigidity (c) Poverty of movements *Consider: (91,* **355-**) Other nervous system diseases NEC; *(254,* **7803**) to *(259,* **7820**) Signs, Symptoms, and Ill-Defined Conditions in Section XVI	332
89	345-	**Epilepsy, all types** *excl.* convulsions, febrile or NOS *(254,* **7803**) *Inclusion in this rubric requires* both *of the following:* (a) Recurrent episodes of altered consciousness of sudden onset with or without tonic or clonic movements (b) Either eyewitness account of the attack of characteristic abnormality of electroencephalogram (EEG)	345

Position no.	ICHPPC code	List of diseases, disorders, and health problems, with inclusion criteria	Comparable ICD-9 codes
90	**346-**	**Migraine** *Inclusion in this rubric requires* one *of the following:* (a) Recurrent episodes of unilateral headache with *one* of the following: (i) Nausea or vomiting (ii) Aura (iii) Neurological disturbance, including visual (iv) Family history of migraine (b) Recurrent bilateral headaches with *three* or more of the above (i to iv) *Consider: (258, **7840**)* Headache	346
91	**355-**	**Other diseases of the nervous system** *incl.* Bell's palsy; benign essential and familial tremor; cerebral palsy; meningitis NEC; Morton's metatarsalgia; peripheral neuropathy (primary and secondary); reaction to lumbar puncture; restless legs syndrome; trigeminal neuralgia *excl.* dementia (*66*, **294-**); effects of head injury on neurological (*332*, **908-**) or psychological (*86*, **316-**) function; post-stroke paralysis (*124*, **438-**); vertebrogenic compression syndromes (*235*, **723-**), (*237*, **721-**), (*239*, **7244**) *Inclusion criteria for this rubric are not listed*	320–331, 333–337, 341–344, 347–359

Diseases of the eye and adnexa

Position no.	ICHPPC code	List of diseases, disorders, and health problems, with inclusion criteria	Comparable ICD-9 codes
92	**3720**	**Conjunctivitis** *incl.* bacterial NOS; allergic *excl.* allergic with rhinorrhea (*145*, **477-**); conjunctivitis proven to be caused by specific organisms (Section I); trachoma (*31*, **136-**); viral conjunctivitis (*18*, **077-**) *Inclusion in this rubric requires:* Inflammation of conjunctivae in the absence of those conditions listed under exclusions	372.0–372.3
93	**3730**	**Stye, hordoleum, chalazion, infected meibomian cyst, blepharitis** *incl.* infection, dermatitis, dermatosis of eyelids *Inclusion in this rubric requires:* Generalized or localized inflammation of the eyelids, including the tarsal glands	373.0–373.2

Position no.	ICHPPC code	List of diseases, disorders, and health problems, with inclusion criteria	Comparable ICD-9 codes
94	367-	**Refractive errors** *excl.* blindness and reduced visual acuity NOS (*98*, **369-**) *Inclusion in this rubric requires:* Visual deficit correctible with an appropriate lens	367
95	—	(*Deleted*)	
96	366-	**Cataract** *Inclusion in this rubric requires:* Opacity of part or all of the optic lens	366
97	365-	**Glaucoma** *incl.* raised intraocular pressure *Inclusion in this rubric requires:* Demonstration of increased intra-ocular pressure or other pathognomonic proof *Consider:* (*99*, **378-**) Other eye diseases	365
98	369-	**Blindness, reduced visual acuity** *excl.* snowblindness, nightblindness (*99*, **378**) *Inclusion in this rubric requires:* **A.** *For blindness—one of the following:* (a) Visual acuity using both eyes of less than 3/60 (20/400) with the best possible correction (b) A defect of visual field in both eyes to 10 degrees or less around central fixation (tunnel vision) **B.** *For reduced visual acuity:* Reduced visual acuity NYD or NOS in one or both eyes	369
99	378-	**Other diseases of the eye** *incl.* arcus senilis; blurred vision; dacryocystitis; diplopia; ectropion; eye pain; iritis; keratitis; night blindness; papilledema; photophobia; pterygium; red eye; retinopathies; snowblindness; spontaneous subconjunctival hemorrhage; strabismus *excl.* foreign body in eye (*330*, **930-**) *Inclusion criteria for this rubric are not listed*	360–364, 368, 370, 371, 372.4–372.9, 373.3–373.9, 374–479

Position no.	ICHPPC code	List of diseases, disorders, and health problems, with inclusion criteria	Comparable ICD-9 codes

Diseases of the ear and mastoid process

100	**3801**	**Otitis externa** *incl.* eczema of external auditory meatus *excl.* boil of external auditory meatus (*207*, **680-**) *Inclusion in this rubric requires:* Inflammation or desquamation of the external auditory canal	380.1, 380.2
101	**3820**	**Acute (suppurative) otitis media, acute myringitis, otitis media NOS** *Inclusion in this rubric requires* one *of the following:* (a) Recent perforation of the tympanic membrane discharging pus (b) Inflamed and bulging tympanic membrane (c) One ear drum is more red than the other (d) Red tympanic membrane, with ear pain (e) Bullae on the tympanic membrane *Consider:* (*102*, **3811**) Non-suppurative otitis media; (*103*, **3815**) Eustachian salpingitis or block; (*107*, **388-**) Chronic suppurative otitis media	382.0, 382.4, 382.9, 384.0
102	**3811**	**Non-suppurative otitis media** *incl.* acute or chronic; 'glue' ear; serous otitis media *Inclusion in this rubric requires* one *of the following:* (a) Visible fluid behind the tympanic membrane, without inflammation (b) Dullness of the tympanic membrane with either retraction or bulging (c) Dullness of the tympanic membrane with related impairment of hearing *Consider:* (*101*, **3820**) Otitis media NOS; (*103*, **3815**) Eustachian salpingitis or block	381.0–381.4
103	**3815**	**Eustachian salpingitis or block** *Inclusion in this rubric requires* both *of the following:* (a) Acute onset of impairment of hearing (b) Discomfort in the ear with shiny normal colored tympanic membrane *Consider:* (*101*, **3820**) Otitis media NOS; (*102*, **3811**) Non-suppurative otitis media	381.5, 381.6

Position no.	ICHPPC code	List of diseases, disorders, and health problems, with inclusion criteria	Comparable ICD-9 codes
104	386-	**Vertiginous syndromes, disorders of the labyrinth and vestibular system** *incl.* benign paroxysmal and positional vertigo; labyrinthitis; Menière's disease; vestibular neuronitis *excl.* giddiness, dizziness NOS (*256*, **7804**) *Inclusion in this rubric requires:* True rotational vertigo	386
105	387-	**Deafness NOS, otosclerosis** *excl.* other specified forms of deafness (other rubrics in this section) *Inclusion in this rubric requires:* Persistent reduction in hearing acuity in one or both ears with normal otoscopic appearance	387, 389, 388.2
106	3804	**Wax in ear canal** *Inclusion in this rubric requires:* Reduction in hearing or discomfort due to wax in ear canal	380.4
107	388-	**Other diseases of ear and mastoid process** *incl.* acoustic trauma; chronic suppurative otitis media; cholesteatoma; ear pain NYD or NOS; mastoiditis; non-traumatic perforation of tympanic membrane; presbyacusis; tinnitus *excl.* deafness NOS (*105*, **387-**); traumatic perforation of the tympanic membrane (*323*, **889-**) *Inclusion criteria for this rubric are not listed*	380.0, 380.3, 380.5, 380.9, 381.7, 381.9, 382.1–382.3, 383, 384.1–384.9, 385, 388 ex. 388.2

Position no.	ICHPPC code	List of diseases, disorders, and health problems, with inclusion criteria	Comparable ICD-9 codes

VII. DISEASES OF THE CIRCULATORY SYSTEM

Diseases of the heart

108   **390-**   **Chronic rheumatic heart disease, acute rheumatic fever, Sydenham's chorea, with or without heart involvement**   390–398

excl. chronic disease of valve or endocardium when not specified as rheumatic, and where rheumatic origin is *not* suggested on clinical grounds (e.g. it *would* be in the following: mitral stenosis, combined disease of mitral and aortic valves, tricuspid valve disease)

Inclusion in this rubric requires:

A. *For chronic rheumatic heart disease*—one *of the following:*

(a) Physical findings consistent with a valve lesion of the heart in a patient with a history of rheumatic fever

(b) Physical findings consistent with mitral stenosis, even in the absence of a history of rheumatic fever, but without any other demonstrable cause

B. *For acute rheumatic fever*—two *major, or* one major and two *minor manifestations,* plus *evidence of preceding streptococcal infection:*

(a) Major manifestations:
  (i) Migratory polyarthritis
  (ii) Carditis
  (iii) Sydenham's chorea
  (iv) Erythema marginatum
  (v) Subcutaneous nodules of recent onset

(b) Minor manifestations:
  (i) Fever
  (ii) Arthralgia
  (iii) Prior history of rheumatic fever or rheumatic heart disease
  (iv) Elevated ESR or positive C-reactive protein
  (v) Prolonged P-R interval on ECG

C. *For Sydenham's chorea, with or without heart involvement*—all *of the following:*

(a) Explosive speech

(b) Hyperactive purposeless writhing movements of face, arms, and legs, which occur while awake (not during sleep) and are usually symmetrical

(c) Muscular weakness

Position no.	ICHPPC code	List of diseases, disorders, and health problems, with inclusion criteria	Comparable ICD-9 codes

109	**410-**	**Acute myocardial infarction, subacute ischemic heart disease**
		Inclusion in this rubric requires:
		A. *For acute myocardial infarction*—two *of the following within 8 weeks of onset:*
		(a) Chest pain characteristic of myocardial ischemia, lasting more than 15 minutes
		(b) Abnormal ST-T changes or Q waves in electrocardiogram
		(c) Elevation of blood cardiac enzymes
		B. *For subacute ischemic heart disease*—both *of the following within 8 weeks of onset:*
		(a) *One* of the following:
		   (i) Severe anginal chest pain at rest lasting over 15 minutes
		   (ii) Recent increased frequency and severity of anginal chest pain
		(b) Does not fulfil criteria for acute myocardial infarction (A above)
		Consider· (*110*, **412-**) Chronic ischemic heart disease
			410–411

110	**412-**	**Chronic ischemic heart disease** *incl.* angina pectoris; aneurysm of heart; asymptomatic ischemic heart disease; cardiosclerosis; healed myocardial infarction; *excl.* atherosclerotic valve disease (*111*, **424-**) *Note:* Requires additional code for hypertension *Inclusion in this rubric requires* one *of the following:* (a) History, ECG, or evidence by radiological technique of old myocardial infarction (b) Chest pain compatible with angina pectoris (c) Demonstration of myocardial ischemia by resting or exercise ECG (d) X-ray evidence of coronary artery narrowing (e) ECG or X-ray evidence of ventricular aneurysm	412–414
111	—	(See after position number 117)	

Position no.	ICHPPC code	List of diseases, disorders, and health problems, with inclusion criteria	Comparable ICD-9 codes

112   **428-**   **Heart failure, right sided or left sided**   428
Note: requires additional code for hypertension or other known cause
Inclusion in the rubric requires three *of the following:*
  (a) Dependent edema
  (b) Raised jugular venous pressure or hepatomegaly in the absence of liver disease
  (c) Signs of pulmonary congestion or pleural effusion
  (d) Enlarged heart
  (e) Dyspnea in the absence of pulmonary disease

113   **4273**   **Atrial fibrillation or flutter**   427.3
Inclusion in this rubric requires one *of the following:*
  (a) Demonstration of characteristic findings by electrocardiogram
  (b) Totally irregular heart rate, with a pulse deficit
Consider: (*263*, **7851**) Palpitations;
(*300*, **7889**) Tachycardia NOS

114   **4270**   **Paroxysmal tachycardia**   427.0–427.2
(Supraventricular, ventricular, or unspecified)
excl. tachycardia NOS (*300*, **7889**)
Inclusion in this rubric requires:
A history of recurrent episodes of rapid heart rate (over 140/min.) with both abrupt onset and termination
Consider: (*263*, **7851**) Palpitations

115   **4276**   **Ectopic beats, all types**   427.6
incl. premature beats, PVB, PNB, PAB
excl. wandering pacemaker (*118*, **429-**)
Inclusion in this rubric requires:
The finding of one or more heart beats which occur at times other than the regular beats of the underlying rhythm
Note: If ectopic beats are frequent (more than 10/min.) an electrocardiogram is suggested to distinguish from other disorders of cardiac rhythm
Consider: (*118*, **429-**) Other heart diseases

Position no.	ICHPPC code	List of diseases, disorders, and health problems, with inclusion criteria	Comparable ICD-9 codes
116	**7852**	(See after position number 264)	
117	**416-**	**Pulmonary heart disease (chronic) cor pulmonale** Inclusion in this rubric requires both of the following: (a) Presence of a chronic disease of the lungs, pulmonary vasculature, or respiratory gas exchange (b) Presence of right ventricular enlargement or right heart failure *Consider: (112, **428-**) Right heart failure*	416
(111)	**424-**	**Diseases of heart valve NOS, NYD, or specified as of non-rheumatic cause** *Inclusion in this rubric requires both of the following:* (a) Absence of criteria for chronic rheumatic heart disease *(108, **390-** A)* (b) Evidence of valvular dysfunction by either characteristic heart murmur alone or by heart murmur plus X-ray or echocardiographic evidence of abnormal valve *Consider: (116, **7852**) Heart murmur NEC or NYD; (121, **402-**) Hypertensive heart disease*	424
118	**429-**	**All other heart disease** *incl.* acute and subacute endocarditis; cardiac arrest; cardiomegaly; cardiomyopathy; disturbances of heart rhythm (other); myocarditis; pericarditis (other than rheumatic) *excl.* hypertensive heart disease *(121, **402-**)* *Inclusion criteria for this rubric are not listed*	420, 421, 422, 423, 425, 426, 427.5, 427.8, 427.9, 429.0, 429.1, 429.2, 429.3

Blood pressure problems

119	**7962**	(See after position numbers 298 and (375), (51), (376))	

Position no.	ICHPPC code	List of diseases, disorders, and health problems, with inclusion criteria	Comparable ICD-9 codes
120	**401-**	**Uncomplicated hypertension, primary or secondary** *incl.* hypertension NOS; labile hypertension *Note:* if secondary hypertension, code for underlying cause *Inclusion in this rubric requires* both *of the following:* (a) *One* of the following: (i) Two or more readings per encounter, taken at two or more encounters, with blood pressures that average over 95 mm Hg diastolic or over 160 mm Hg systolic in adult patients (ii) Two or more readings at a single encounter with an average diastolic blood pressure of 120 mm Hg or more (b) Absence of evidence of secondary involvement of heart, kidney, or brain due to hypertension *Consider:* (*119*, **7962**) elevated blood pressure—for diastolic blood pressure range of 90 to 95 mm Hg or systolic blood pressure range of 140 to 160 mm Hg, or other casual raised blood pressure readings. For children, consult appropriate pediatric blood pressure tables *Consider:* (*121*, **402-**) Hypertension with complications	401, pt. 405
121	**402-**	**Hypertension, primary or secondary with involvement of target organs** *incl.* involvement of heart, kidney, or brain (Note: may code the effect as well) *Inclusion in this rubric requires* both *of the following:* (a) Blood pressure levels as defined in rubric (*120*, **401-**) (b) Abnormalities of the heart (enlargement, failure), kidney (albuminuria, azotemia) or brain (abnormalities of fundus, stroke) attributed to hypertension	401.0, 402–404, pt. 405, 437.2
122	—	(*Deleted*)	

Position no.	ICHPPC code	List of diseases, disorders, and health problems, with inclusion criteria	Comparable ICD-9 codes

Diseases of the vascular system

| 123 | 435- | **Transient cerebral ischemia** | 435 |

incl. transient ischemic attack (TIA)
Inclusion in this rubric requires all *of the following:*
(a) Symptoms of transient (less than 24 hours) hypofunction of the brain, with sudden onset
(b) Without sequelae
(c) Exclusion of migraine, migraine equivalent, or epilepsy

| 124 | 438- | **Other cerebrovascular disease** | 430–434, 436–438, ex. 437.2 |

incl. all types of stroke; post-stroke paralysis; subacute and chronic cerebrovascular disease
Inclusion in this rubric requires:
Signs and symptoms of a disturbance of cerebral function, presumed of vascular origin, lasting more than 24 hours or causing death

| 125 | 440- | **Atherosclerosis, except of heart, brain, gut, kidneys, or lung** | 440 |

excl. when causing arterial blockage (*126,* **443-**)
Inclusion in this rubric requires both *of the following:*
(a) Evidence of calcification by palpation or X-ray of an artery (other than those of heart, brain, gut, kidneys, or lung)
(b) Absence of evidence of ischemia

Position no.	ICHPPC code	List of diseases, disorders, and health problems, with inclusion criteria	Comparable ICD-9 codes
126	**443-**	**Other arterial obstruction and peripheral vascular disease**	443, 444

incl. arterial blocks, other; intermittent claudication; Raynaud's phenomenon
excl. aneurysm (*132*, **459-**); occlusion of retinal artery (*99*, **378-**); occlusion of coronary arteries (*109*, **410-**); occlusion of cerebral arteries (*123*, **435-**), (*124*, **438-**); occlusion of pulmonary arteries (*127*, **415-**); occlusion of mesenteric arteries (*167*, **579-**); occlusion of renal arteries (*174*, **598-**); gangrene (*300*, **7889**); chilblains (*377*, **994-**)
Inclusion in this rubric requires one *of the following:*
  (a) Signs or symptoms of tissue ischemia due to obstruction of an artery, excluding arteries of the brain, heart, gut, kidney, and lung
  (b) Investigative evidence of arterial obstruction, excluding arteries of the brain, heart, gut, kidney, and lung

| *127* | **415-** | **Pulmonary embolism and infarction** | 415 |

Inclusion in this rubric requires one *of the following:*
  (a) Sudden onset of dyspnea of tachycardia and the presence of *one* of the following:
    (i) Clinical or X-ray evidence of pulmonary infarction
    (ii) ECG evidence of acute right ventricular strain
  (b) Demonstration of regional pulmonary ischemia on lung scan, in the absence of other diseases capable of producing these changes
  (c) Evidence of filling defects or pulmonary artery occlusion by angiography
Consider: (*269*, **7860**) Dyspnea

Position no.	ICHPPC code	List of diseases, disorders, and health problems, with inclusion criteria	Comparable ICD-9 codes

128	**451-**	**Phlebitis and thrombophlebitis**
		 incl. deep vein thrombosis; phlebothrombosis; portal thrombosis
		 excl. cerebral thrombosis (*124*, **438-**); thrombophlebitis in pregnancy (*202*, **648-**) or in puerperium (*206*, **670-**)
		 Inclusion in this rubric requires:
		 A. *For superficial phlebitis or thrombophlebitis (phlebothrombosis):*
		 Signs of inflammation along a superficial vein
		 B. *For deep vein thrombosis—one of the following:*
		 (a) Demonstration of thrombosis by phlebography or ultrasound
		 (b) *All* of the following:
		   (i) Swelling of extremity
		   (ii) Increased warmth of extremity
		   (iii) Linear tenderness over the course of a vein or a positive Homan's sign
		 Consider: (*286*, **7295**) Pain and other symptoms referrable to a limb
		 C. *For portal vein thrombosis:*
		 Thrombosis demonstrated by radiological technique or at surgery
			451–453

129	**454-**	**Varicose veins of legs, with or without ulcer or eczema** *incl.* venous insufficiency; venous stasis *Inclusion in this rubric requires* one *of the following:* (a) Presence of dilated superficial veins in lower extremities (b) Demonstration of valve incompetence	454
130	**455-**	**Hemorrhoids** *incl.* residual hemorrhoidal skin tags; thrombosed external piles (perianal hematoma) *Inclusion in this rubric requires* one *of the following:* (a) Visualization of varicosities of the venous plexus of the anus or canal (b) Tender, painful, blue-coloured localized swelling of acute onset, in the perianal area (c) Skin tags in the perianal area *Consider:* (*163*, **5646**) Anal pain NOS	455

Position no.	ICHPPC code	List of diseases, disorders, and health problems, with inclusion criteria	Comparable ICD-9 codes
131	**4580**	**Postural hypotension, low blood pressure** *Inclusion in this rubric requires* both *of the following:* (a) Signs or symptoms of cerebrovascular insufficiency (dizziness, syncope) on changing from the supine to the upright position (b) A fall in mean blood pressure of 15 mm Hg on two or more occasions when changing from the supine to the upright position *Consider: (338,* **V70-***)* Normal variation	458
132	**459-**	**Other diseases of peripheral blood-vessels** *incl.* aneurysm; esophageal varices; lymphangitis; polyarteritis nodosa; temporal arteritis; varicocele *Inclusion criteria for this rubric are not listed*	441, 442, 446–448, 456, 457, 459

Position no.	ICHPPC code	List of diseases, disorders, and health problems, with inclusion criteria	Comparable ICD-9 codes

VIII. DISEASES OF THE RESPIRATORY SYSTEM

133	**460-**	**Upper respiratory tract infection, acute** *incl.* cold; nasopharyngitis; pharyngitis; rhinitis *excl.* that of proven specific origin (Section I); influenza *(139,* **487-**); viral pharyngoconjunctivitis *(18,* **077-**) *Inclusion in this rubric requires* both *of the following:* (a) Evidence of acute inflammation of nasal or pharyngeal mucosa (b) Absence of criteria for more specifically defined acute respiratory infection classified in this section	460, 462, 465

134	**461-**	**Sinusitis, acute and chronic**
		Inclusion in this rubric requires one *of the following:*
		(a) Pus obtained directly from sinus
		(b) *Two* of the following:
		   (i) Purulent nasal or postnasal discharge, or previous medically treated episodes of sinusitis
		   (ii) Tenderness over one or more sinuses, or deep-seated aching facial pain aggravated by dependency of head
		   (iii) Radiological evidence of sinusitis or opacity on transillumination
		Consider: (133, **460-**) Upper respiratory tract infection; *(258,* **7840**) Headache or pain in face NOS; *(145,* **477-**) Allergic rhinitis
			461, 473

135	**463-**	**Tonsillitis, acute, quinsy (peritonsillar abscess)** *excl.* that of proven streptococcal origin *(7,* **034**) *Inclusion in this rubric requires* four *of the following:* (a) Sore throat (b) Reddening of tonsil(s) more than the posterior pharyngeal wall (c) Pus on tonsil(s) (d) Swelling of the tonsil(s) (e) Enlarged tender regional lymph nodes (f) Fever *Consider: (133,* **460-**) Acute upper respiratory tract infection; *(17,* **075-**) Infectious mononucleosis	463, 475

Position no.	ICHPPC code	List of diseases, disorders, and health problems, with inclusion criteria	Comparable ICD-9 codes
136	**474-**	**Hypertrophy and chronic infection of tonsils and adenoids**	474

Inclusion in this rubric requires:
A. *For hypertrophy of tonsils—both of the following:*
(a) Enlargement of the tonsils sufficient to cause *one* of the following:
   (i) Tonsils touch in midline
   (ii) Respiratory difficulty
   (iii) Difficulty in swallowing
(b) No acute respiratory infection within the previous 4 weeks
B. *For chronic infection of the tonsils:*
More than 4 medically diagnosed episodes of acute tonsillitis in 2 years (or 3 in 1 year)
C. *For hypertrophy of adenoids—two of the following:*
(a) Mouth-breathing
(b) Demonstration of enlarged adenoids
(c) At least 4 episodes of medically diagnosed otitis media in 2 years (or 3 in 1 year)
Consider: (300, **7889***)* Other symptoms, signs and ill-defined conditions

Position no.	ICHPPC code	List of diseases, disorders, and health problems, with inclusion criteria	Comparable ICD-9 codes
137	**464-**	**Laryngitis and tracheitis, acute**	464

incl. croup, epiglottitis
Inclusion in this rubric requires:
A. *For laryngitis, acute, croup and epiglottitis—one of the following:*
(a) Hoarseness
(b) Stridor
(c) Visibly red epiglottis
B. *For tracheitis, acute—both of the following:*
(a) Persistent deep dry painful cough (barking in children)
(b) Absence of abnormal chest signs
Consider: (133, **460-***)* Upper respiratory tract infection

Position no.	ICHPPC code	List of diseases, disorders, and health problems, with inclusion criteria	Comparable ICD-9 codes
138	466-	**Bronchitis, bronchiolitis, acute**	466, 490

incl. bronchitis NOS; tracheobronchitis
Inclusion in this rubric requires both *of the following:*
(a) Cough
(b) Scattered or generalized abnormal chest signs—wheeze, coarse or moist sounds
Note: Bronchiolitis in infants may be present as dyspnea and obstructive emphysema without wheeze, moist sounds, fever, or sputum
Consider: (*133*, **460-**) Upper respiratory tract infection; (*144*, **493-**) Asthma; (*269*, **7860**) Wheezing; (*270*, **7862**) Cough

Position no.	ICHPPC code	List of diseases, disorders, and health problems, with inclusion criteria	Comparable ICD-9 codes
139	487-	**Influenza, without pneumonia**	487 ex. 487.0

incl. influenza-like illness
excl. gastric flu (*2*, **009-**); influenzal pneumonia (*140*, **486-**); viral infection NOS (*20*, **0799**)
Inclusion in this rubric requires one *of the following:*
(a) Viral culture or serological evidence of influenza virus infection
(b) Influenza epidemic, plus *four* of the criteria in (c)
(c) *Six* of the following:
  (i) Sudden onset (within 12 hours)
  (ii) Cough
  (iii) Rigors or chills
  (iv) Fever
  (v) Prostration and weakness
  (vi) Myalgia, widespread aches and pains
  (vii) No significant respiratory physical signs other than redness of nasal mucous membrane and throat
  (viii) Influenza in close contacts
Consider: (*133*, **460-**) Upper respiratory tract infection, acute; (*20*, **0799**) Viral infection NOS

Position no.	ICHPPC code	List of diseases, disorders, and health problems, with inclusion criteria	Comparable ICD-9 codes

140	**486-**	**Pneumonia**
		incl. bacterial and viral pneumonia; influenzal pneumonia
		excl. aspiration pneumonia (*147*, **519-**)
		Inclusion in this rubric requires:
		Evidence of pulmonary consolidation shown by *one* of the following:
		(a) Typical X-ray appearance
		(b) Clinical signs of *three* of the following:
		   (i) Diminished air entry
		   (ii) Dullness to percussion
		   (iii) Bronchial breath sounds
		   (iv) Fine crepitations
		   (v) Increased vocal fremitus and resonance
		Consider: (*138*, **466-**) Bronchitis and bronchiolitis, acute; (*147*, **519-**) Other respiratory system disease
			480–486, 487.0

141	**5110**	**Pleurisy, all types, except tuberculosis**
		excl. pleural effusion NOS (*5*, **5119**)
		Inclusion in this rubric requires one of the following:
		(a) Histological evidence of inflammation on pleural biopsy
		(b) Cytological or bacteriological evidence of inflammation in the pleural fluid
		(c) Pleuritic pain, accompanied by *one* of the following:
		   (i) Pleural friction rub on auscultation
		   (ii) Either clinical or investigative evidence of pleural exudate
			511.0–511.8

(*5*)	**5119**	**Pleural effusion NOS** *Inclusion in this rubric requires:* The painless accumulation of excessive fluid in the pleural cavity (as shown clinically or by investigation), where *one* of the following applies: (a) No cause has yet been found (b) Inflammatory causes have been excluded	511.9

Position no.	ICHPPC code	List of diseases, disorders, and health problems, with inclusion criteria	Comparable ICD-9 codes
142	**491-**	**Chronic bronchitis, bronchiectasis** *Inclusion in this rubric requires* both *of the following:* (a) Cough with purulent sputum on most days for at least 3 months in each of at least 2 years (b) Scattered rales or rhonchi on auscultation of the chest during these episodes *Consider: (138,* **466-**) Bronchitis NOS; *(143,* **492-**) Emphysema and COPD	491, 494
143	**492-**	**Emphysema, chronic obstructive pulmonary disease (COPD, cold)** *excl.* bronchiectasis *(142,* **491-**) *Inclusion in this rubric requires* one *of the following:* (a) X-ray evidence of emphysema (b) Airway obstruction, not relieved or only partially relieved, by bronchodilators at pulmonary function test (c) *Both* of the following: (i) Dyspnea on exertion (ii) Barrel-shaped, hyper-resonant, poorly moving chest with reduced breath sounds on auscultation	492, 496
144	**493-**	**Asthma** *Inclusion in this rubric requires:* Recurrent episodes of acute bronchial obstruction with *one* of the following: (a) Pulmonary function tests showing variable obstruction, relieved by bronchodilators (b) *Two* of the following: (i) Wheeze (ii) Dry cough (iii) Prolonged expiratory phase of respiratory cycle *Consider: (138,* **466-**) Bronchitis and bronchiolitis; *(143,* **492-**) Emphysema, COPD; *(269,* **7860**) Wheezing; *(270,* **7862**) Cough	493
145	**477-**	**Hay fever, allergic rhinitis** *excl.* nasal polyps *(147,* **519-**) *Inclusion in this rubric requires* three *of the following on a chronic or seasonal basis:* (a) Sneezing (b) Nasal obstruction (c) Clear nasal discharge (d) Watering eyes (e) Edema of the nasal mucosa	477

Position no.	ICHPPC code	List of diseases, disorders, and health problems, with inclusion criteria	Comparable ICD-9 codes
146	**4781**	**Boil or abscess in nose** *excl.* boil of skin of nose (*207*, **680**) *As defined in the diagnostic title*	pt. 478.1
147	**519-**	**Other diseases of respiratory system** *incl.* allergic pneumonitis; chronic URTI; deviated nasal septum; empyema; lung complications of other diseases; other diseases of larynx; pneumoconiosis; pneumothorax; *excl.* cystic fibrosis affecting lungs (*57*, **279-**); lung cancer (*33*, **162-**) *Inclusion criteria for this rubric are not listed*	470–472, 476, 478 ex. pt. 478.1, 495, 500–510, 512–519

IX. DISEASES OF THE DIGESTIVE SYSTEM

148   **520-**   **Diseases of the teeth and supporting structures**   520–526
incl. caries; dental abscess; disorders of temporomandibular joint; gingivitis; teething
Inclusion criteria for this rubric are not listed

149   **528-**   **Diseases of the mouth, tongue and salivary glands**   527–529
incl. angular cheilosis; apthous ulcer; effect of dentures; glossitis; mucocele; salivary calculus; stomatitis
excl. herpes simplex (*11,* **054-**); mumps (*16,* **072-**)
Inclusion criteria for this rubric are not listed

150   **530-**   **Diseases of esophagus**   530
incl. esophagitis
excl. cancer of esophagus (*32,* **151**); esophageal varices (*132,* **459-**)
Inclusion criteria for this rubric are not listed

151   **532-**   **Duodenal ulcer,** with or without complications   532
Inclusion in this rubric requires one *of the following:*
(a) Characteristic X-ray findings
(b) Characteristic endoscopy findings
(c) Exacerbation of symptoms in a patient with a previously proven duodenal ulcer
Consider: (*150,* **530-**) Esophagitis; (*153,* **536-**) Indigestion NOS; (*275,* **7871**) Heartburn

152   **533-**   **Other peptic ulcers**   531, 533, 534
incl. gastric, gastrojejunal, marginal, and peptic ulcer NOS
Inclusion in this rubric requires one *of the following:*
(a) Characteristic X-ray findings
(b) Characteristic endoscopy findings
(c) Exacerbation of symptoms in a patient with a previously proven ulcer
Consider: (*150,* **530-**) Esophagitis; (*153,* **536-**) Indigestion NOS; (*275,* **7871**) Heartburn

Position no.	ICHPPC code	List of diseases, disorders, and health problems, with inclusion criteria	Comparable ICD-9 codes
153	**536-**	**Disorders of stomach function and other diseases of stomach and duodenum** *incl.* duodenitis; dyspepsia; gastritis (incl. alcoholic); indigestion NOS *excl.* infective gastritis or enteritis (*1*, **008-**) (*2*, **009-**) *Inclusion in this rubric requires:* Meal-related epigastric pain or discomfort *Consider:* (*150*, **530-**) Esophagitis; (*274*, **7870**) Vomiting, nausea; (*275*, **7871**) Heartburn; (*278*, **7873**) Gas problems (wind); (*279*, **7890**) Abdominal pain	535–537
154	**540-**	**Appendicitis, all types** *Inclusion in this rubric requires:* Inflammation of the appendix demonstrated at surgery or on histology *Consider:* (*279*, **7890**) Abdominal pain	540–542
155	**550-**	**Inguinal hernia**—with or without obstruction *Inclusion in this rubric requires* both *of the following:* (a) Swelling in the inguinal region (b) *One* of the following: (i) Transmitted impulse with cough (ii) Enlargement on straining (iii) Reducible into the abdomen (iv) Intestinal obstruction	550
156	**551-**	**Hiatus hernia, diaphragmatic hernia** *Inclusion in this rubric requires:* Characteristic findings on X-ray, endoscopy, intraluminal pressure studies, or at surgery *Consider:* (*150*, **530-**) Esophagitis; (*275*, **7871**) Heartburn	551.3, 552.3, 553.3
157	**553-**	**Other abdominal hernias** *incl.* femoral, incisional, umbilical *Inclusion in this rubric requires demonstration at surgery or* both *of the following:* (a) Swelling in the specified area (b) *One* of the following: (i) Transmitted impulse with cough (ii) Enlargement on straining (iii) Reducible into the abdomen (iv) Intestinal obstruction	551–553 (ex. 551.3, 552.3, 553.3)

Position no.	ICHPPC code	List of diseases, disorders, and health problems, with inclusion criteria	Comparable ICD-9 codes
158	**562-**	**Diverticular disease of intestines** *incl.* diverticulitis; diverticulosis *Inclusion in this rubric requires* one *of the following:* (a) X-ray demonstration of diverticula (b) Demonstration of diverticula at surgery (c) *All* of the following in an adult: (i) Acute abdominal pain (ii) Palpable tender descending or sigmoid colon (iii) Fever *Consider:* (*159,* **558-**) Irritable bowel syndrome; (*279,* **7890**) Abdominal pain	562
159	**558-**	**Irritable bowel syndrome (colospasm, spastic colon, mucous colitis) and other non-infective, non-ulcerative disorders of the intestines** *incl.* allergic, dietetic, and toxic gastroenteritis and colitis; diarrhea NOS, presumed to be non-infective *excl.* intestinal disease which is either proven or presumed to be of infective origin (*1,* **008-**), (*2,* **009-**); psychogenic diarrhea (*71,* **3001**); regional enteritis (*160,* **555-**); vascular insufficiency of gut (*167,* **579-**) *Inclusion criteria are not listed for part of this rubric* *For optional hierarchy, inclusion in this rubric requires:* **A.** *For irritable bowel syndrome*—both *of the following:* (a) Continuous or intermittent abdominal pain and variable bowel pattern for over 3 months (b) *One* of the following: (i) Increased gas (ii) Tender and palpable colon (iii) History of mucus without blood in stool *Consider:* (*160,* **555-**) Crohn's disease, ulcerative colitis; (*161,* **5640**) constipation **B.** *For other disorders*—*inclusion criteria for this part of the rubric are not listed*	558, 564.1, 564.5

Position no.	ICHPPC code	List of diseases, disorders, and health problems, with inclusion criteria	Comparable ICD-9 codes
160	555-	**Chronic enteritis, ulcerative colitis, Crohn's disease** *Inclusion in this rubric requires:* Characteristic endoscopic, radiological, or histological findings for these conditions *Consider: (159,* **558-**) Mucous colitis; (*164,* **5693**) Bleeding per rectum; (*279,* **7890**) Abdominal pain	555, 556
161	**5640**	**Constipation** *excl.* fecal impaction (*167,* **579-**) *Inclusion in this rubric requires* two *of the following:* (a) Hard stools (b) Decreased frequency of stools (c) Difficult evacuation or incomplete emptying of rectum	564.0
162	565-	**Anal fissure and fistula, perianal abscess** *Inclusion in this rubric requires:* **A.** *For anal fissure—the following:* Visible or palpable splitting of mucosa at the anal mucocutaneous junction *Consider:* (*163,* **5646**) Anal pain NOS **B.** *For anal fistula—one of the following:* (a) Demonstration of abnormal channel between skin surface and anal canal (b) History of healed perianal abscess and presence of an external draining skin ostium **C.** *For perianal abscess—the following:* A hard or fluctuant, tender localized perianal swelling, presumed or proven to contain pus	565, 566
163	**5646**	**Rectal and anal pain NOS** *incl.* anal spasm; proctalgia fugax; proctitis NOS *As defined in the diagnostic title*	564.6, pt. 569.4
164	**5693**	**Bleeding per rectum NOS** *excl.* (gastro)intestinal hemorrhage NOS (*276,* **578-**); hemorrhoids (*130,* **455-**) *Inclusion in this rubric requires:* The above symptom(s), without additional criteria needed for inclusion in other rubrics	569.3
(*276*)	**578-**	**Hematemesis, melena** *incl.* (gastro)intestinal hemorrhage NOS *Inclusion in this rubric requires* one *of the following, in the absence of known cause:* (a) Vomiting of blood (b) Passage of black stools from the rectum (c) Demonstration of occult blood in the stool	578

Position no.	ICHPPC code	List of diseases, disorders, and health problems, with inclusion criteria	Comparable ICD-9 codes
165	**571-**	**Cirrhosis and other liver diseases** *excl.* viral hepatitis (*15*, **070-**) *Inclusion criteria are not listed for part of this rubric* *For optional hierarchy, inclusion in this rubric requires:* **A.** *For cirrhosis*—one *of the following:* (a) Diagnostic liver biopsy (b) *Both* of the following: (i) Chronic (more than 3 months) smooth, firm, nontender enlargement of the liver—or abnormal liver function tests, or clinical evidence of liver failure (ii) History of chronic (more than 1 year) heavy alcohol intake, or of other substances capable of causing cirrhosis **B.** *For other liver diseases—inclusion criteria for this part of the rubric are not listed*	570–573

Position no.	ICHPPC code	List of diseases, disorders, and health problems, with inclusion criteria	Comparable ICD-9 codes
166	574-	**Cholecystitis, cholelithiasis, cholangitis and other diseases of the gallbladder and biliary tract**	574–576

166 574- **Cholecystitis, cholelithiasis, cholangitis and other diseases of the gallbladder and biliary tract** 574–576

Inclusion criteria are not listed for part of this rubric

For optional hierarchy, inclusion in this rubric requires:

A. *For acute cholecystitis—one of the following:*
(a) Demonstration of typical pathology at surgery
(b) *Both* of the following:
   (i) Localized right upper quadrant tenderness
   (ii) *Two* of the following:
      1. Right upper quadrant abdominal pain
      2. Jaundice
      3. Fever
      4. History of gall stones

B. *For cholelithiasis—the following:*
X-ray, ultrasound, or surgical demonstration of gall stones

C. *For acute biliary colic—both of the following:*
(a) Acute colicky right upper quadrant abdominal pain with a duration of less than 24 hours, without fever
(b) *One* of the following:
   (i) Jaundice
   (ii) Right upper quadrant abdominal tenderness
   (iii) History of gall stones

D. *For other diseases—inclusion criteria for this part of the rubric are not listed*

167 579- **Other diseases of the digestive system**
incl. dumping syndrome; functional results of gastro-intestinal surgery; ileus; intussuception; intestinal obstruction; malabsorption syndrome; mesenteric vascular insufficiency and block; pancreatic diseases; rectal polyp; secondary megacolon; sprue
excl. malignant disease (*32*, **151-**)
Inclusion criteria for this rubric are not listed

543, 557, 560,
564.2–564.4,
564.7–564.9, 567, 568,
569 ex. 569.3,
pt. 569.4, 577, 579

Position no.	ICHPPC code	List of diseases, disorders, and health problems, with inclusion criteria	Comparable ICD-9 codes

X. DISEASES OF THE GENITOURINARY TRACT

Diseases of the urinary system

168   **580-**   **Glomerulonephritis, acute and chronic**   580–583
incl. nephrosis
Inclusion in this rubric requires:
A. *For acute glomerulonephritis
(nephrosis)—one of the following:*
(a) Typical histological appearance
(b) *Three* of the following:
    (i) Proteinuria
    (ii) Painless hematuria
    (iii) Hypertension
    (iv) Generalized edema
    (v) Hypoalbuminemia
B. *For chronic glomerulonephritis—one of the
following:*
(a) Typical histological appearance
(b) *Four* of the following:
    (i) History of acute glomerulonephritis
    (ii) Proteinuria
    (iii) Decreased renal function
    (iv) Generalized edema
    (v) Microscopic hematuria or cellular or
        waxy casts
    (vi) Hypertension

169   **5901**   **Pyelonephritis and pyelitis, acute**   590.1, 590.3, 590.8,
incl. kidney infection NOS   590.9
excl. pyelonephritis, chronic (*174*, **598-**); in
pregnancy or puerperium (*198*, **6466**)
Inclusion in this rubric requires both *of the
following:*
(a) *Two* of the following:
    (i) Flank pain
    (ii) Fever
    (iii) Renal tenderness
    (iv) Dysuria
(b) Urine culture demonstrating more than
    100 000 bacterial colonies per ml of freshly
    voided midstream urine after washing of
    genitalia
Consider: (*170*, **595-**) Urinary infection NOS;
(*279*, **7890**) Flank pain

Position no.	ICHPPC code	List of diseases, disorders, and health problems, with inclusion criteria	Comparable ICD-9 codes

170	**595-**	**Cystitis and urinary infection NOS**
		 incl. asymptomatic bacteriuria
		 excl. in pregnancy or puerperium (*198,* **6466**)
		 Inclusion in this rubric requires one *of the following:*
		 (a) Urine culture demonstrating more than 100000 bacterial colonies per ml of freshly voided midstream urine after washing of genitalia
		 (b) *All* of the following:
		    (i) Dysuria or indwelling urinary catheter
		    (ii) Demonstration of significant numbers of pus cells or bacteria in freshly voided midstream urine by microscopy
		    (iii) Absence of balanitis, urethritis, or vaginitis
		 Consider: (*172,* **597-**) Urethritis; (*280,* **7881**) Dysuria; (*283,* **7884**) frequency of urination; (*298,* **791-**) Abnormal urine test
			595, 599.0

171	**592-**	**Urinary calculus,** all types and sites
		 Inclusion in this rubric requires one *of the following:*
		 (a) Passage of calculus
		 (b) Radiological evidence of calculus
		 (c) Ureteral colicky pain and *one* of the following:
		    (i) Hematuria
		    (ii) History of stone in the past
		 Consider: (*300,* **7889**) renal colic; (*373,* **5997**) Hematuria
			592, 594

Position no.	ICHPPC code	List of diseases, disorders, and health problems, with inclusion criteria	Comparable ICD-9 codes
172	**597-**	**Urethritis (non-venereal) NEC, NOS**	597

172   **597-**   **Urethritis (non-venereal) NEC, NOS**   597
incl. meatitis, urethral syndrome
Inclusion criteria are not listed for part of this rubric
For optional hierarchy, inclusion in this rubric requires:
A. *For urethritis*—both *of the following:*
(a) Urethral discharge, presumed not to be sexually transmitted
(b) Negative laboratory tests for gonococcus
B. *For meatitis:*
Inflammation of external urinary meatus, presumed not to be sexually transmitted
C. *For urethral syndrome*—both *of the following:*
(a) Frequency, burning, pain, or urgency on urination without urethral discharge
(b) Urine culture with less than 100000 bacterial colonies per ml of freshly voided midstream urine after washing of genitalia without recent antibiotic therapy
D. *For other inflammatory disease of the urethra:*
Inclusion criteria for this part of the rubric are not listed
Consider: (*23,* **098-**) Gonorrhea; (*280,* **7881**) Dysuria; (*372,* **0994**) Nonspecific urethritis; (*300,* **7889**) Urethral discharge NYD

173   **5936**   **Orothostatic albuminuria (postural proteinuria)**   593.6
Inclusion in this rubric requires all *of the following:*
(a) Albuminuria following ambulation
(b) No albuminuria following lying down overnight recumbency
(c) No evidence of renal disease

(*373*)   **5997**   **Hematuria NOS**   599.7
Inclusion in this rubric requires:
Microscopic, macroscopic, or positive chemical test for blood in urine, in the absence of a specific etiology

174   **598-**   **Other diseases of the kidney, ureter, bladder and urethra**   584–589, 590.0, 590.2, 591, 593 ex. 593.6, 596, 598, 599.1–599.6, 599.8–599.9
incl. chronic pyelonephritis; hydronephrosis; renal failure; urethral caruncle; urethral stricture
excl. malignant disease (*37,* **188-**)
Inclusion criteria for this rubric are not listed

Position no.	ICHPPC code	List of diseases, disorders, and health problems, with inclusion criteria	Comparable ICD-9 codes

Diseases of the male genital organs

175   **600-**   **Benign prostatic hypertrophy**   600
incl. fibroma; hyperplasia; median bar of prostate;
prostatic obstruction NOS
*Inclusion in this rubric requires both of the
following:*
(a) Enlarged, smooth, firm prostate
demonstrated by palpation, cystoscopy, or
cystography
(b) No evidence of prostatic carcinoma
Consider: (*300,* **7889**) Retention of urine

176   **601-**   **Prostatitis, seminal vesiculitis**   601, 608.0
*Inclusion in this rubric requires two of the
following:*
(a) Tenderness of prostate or seminal vesicles
to palpation
(b) Increased white cells (more than 15/hpf) in
prostatic fluid following massage
(c) *One* of the following:
(i) Perineal fullness or pain
(ii) Low back pain
(iii) Dysuria

177   **603-**   **Hydrocele**   603
*Inclusion in this rubric requires both of the
following:*
(a) Non-tender fluctuant swelling surrounding
the testes or spermatic cord
(b) Transillumination of the swelling

178   **604-**   **Orchitis, epididymitis**   604
excl. gonococcal (*23,* **098**); mumps (*16,* **072-**);
tuberculosis (*4,* **011**)
*Inclusion in this rubric requires both of the
following:*
(a) Both swelling and tenderness of testes or
epididymis
(b) Absence of a specific etiology (mumps,
gonococcal, tuberculosis, trauma, or
torsion)
Consider: (*180,* **607-**) Torsion of the testis

Position no.	ICHPPC code	List of diseases, disorders, and health problems, with inclusion criteria	Comparable ICD-9 codes
179	605-	**Redundant prepuce, phimosis, balanitis** *Inclusion in this rubric requires:* **A.** *For redundant prepuce:* Excessive length of prepuce, with inability to retract over the glans penis **B.** *For phimosis:* Tightness of the prepuce which prevents retraction over the glans penis **C.** *For balanitis:* Signs of inflammation of the prepuce or glans penis	605, 607.1
180	607-	**Other diseases of the male genitalia** *incl.* spermatocele; torsion of the testis *Inclusion criteria for this rubric are not listed*	602, 607 ex. 607.1, 608, ex. 608.0

Diseases of the breast

181	610-	**Chronic cystic disease of the breast (fibroadenosis) and other benign mammary dysplasias**
		 Inclusion in this rubric requires one *of the following:*
		 (a) Characteristic histological appearance on breast biopsy
		 (b) Aspirate compatible with chronic benign cystic disease
		 (c) *All* of the following:
		    (i) Multiple tender lumps
		    (ii) Variation in size of lumps with menstrual cycle
		    (iii) No clinical evidence of malignancy
		 Consider: (182, **611***)* Lump in breast NOS
			610

182	611-	**Other disorders of breast** *incl.* fat necrosis; galactorhea (not associated with childbirth); gynecomastia; lump in breast NOS; mastodynia; nipple discharge; non-puerperal breast abscess *Inclusion criteria for this rubric are not listed* *Consider: (205,* **676-***)* if in puerperium or during lactation	611

Position no.	ICHPPC code	List of diseases, disorders, and health problems, with inclusion criteria	Comparable ICD-9 codes

Diseases of the female genital organs

183   **614-**   **Pelvic inflammatory disease**   614, 615
incl. endometritis; oophoritis; salpingitis
excl. venereal diseases (*22*, **090-**), (*23*, **098-**), (*31*, **136-**)
Inclusion in this rubric requires one *of the following:*
(a) Demonstration of inflamed Fallopian tube(s) at surgery or laparoscopy
(b) *Three* of the following:
  (i) Lower abdominal pain
  (ii) Tenderness of uterus or adnexa by palpation
  (iii) Elevated ESR, WBC, or fever
  (iv) Past history of pelvic inflammatory disease
Consider: (*194*, **629-**) Pelvic congestion syndrome

184   **622-**   **Cervicitis, cervical erosion, and other**   616.0, 622
abnormalities of the cervix
incl. cervical dysplasia; cervical leukoplakia; mucous cervical polyp; old laceration
excl. abnormalities of cervix in pregnancy, childbirth, and puerperium (*202*, **648-**), (*204*, **661-**), (*206*, **670-**); adenomatous polyp (*43*, **218-**); abnormal Pap smear NOS (*376*, **7950**)
As defined in the diagnostic title

185   **6161**   **Vaginitis NOS, vulvitis**   616.1
excl. urogenital candidiasis—proven (*26*, **1121**); urogenital trichomoniasis—proven (*27*, **1310**); senile vaginitis (*187*, **627-**); leukorrhea (non-infective), fluor vaginalis (*194*, **629-**)
Inclusion in this rubric requires:
A. *For vaginitis NOS*—all *of the following:*
(a) Vaginal discharge
(b) Inflammation of vaginal wall
(c) Absence of proof for specific causes of vaginitis
B. *For vulvitis*—both *of the following:*
(a) Inflammation of the vulva
(b) Absence of proof for specific causes of vulvitis

Position no.	ICHPPC code	List of diseases, disorders, and health problems, with inclusion criteria	Comparable ICD-9 codes
186	**618-**	**Uterovaginal prolapse** *incl.* cystocele; rectocele; stress incontinence NOS *Inclusion in this rubric requires* one *of the following:* (a) Abnormal descent of the cervix or bulge of the anterior or posterior wall of the vagina, on straining at vaginoscopy (b) Involuntary loss of urine on straining or with activity	618, 625.6
187	**627-**	**Menopausal symptoms (climacteric)** *incl.* senile vaginitis; postmenopausal bleeding *Inclusion in this rubric requires:* **A.** *For menopausal symptoms—*both *of the following:* (a) Hot flushes (b) Occurrence near or after age of expected ovarian failure, or following surgical removal (or destruction by radiation) of ovaries **B.** *For senile vaginitis—*both *of the following:* (a) Thin, dry, pale, tight, friable vaginal mucosa (b) Occurrence near or after the age of expected ovarian failure, or following surgical removal (or destruction by radiation) of ovaries **C.** *For postmenopausal bleeding:* Vaginal bleeding following a six-month period of amenorrhea after the expected time of ovarian failure	627

188	**6254**	**Premenstrual tension syndromes**
		 Inclusion in this rubric requires all *of the following:*
		 (a) *One* of the following:
		   (i) Edema
		   (ii) Breast tenderness
		   (iii) Headache
		   (iv) Irritability
		   (v) Mood changes
		   (vi) Peripheral neuropathy
		 (b) Cyclic recurrence during the second half of the menstrual cycle
		 (c) Symptoms disappear at or shortly after onset of menses
			625.4

Position no.	ICHPPC code	List of diseases, disorders, and health problems, with inclusion criteria	Comparable ICD-9 codes
(*374*)	6250	**Vaginismus, dyspareunia in the female** not specified as psychogenic *Inclusion in this rubric requires* both *of the following:* (a) Vaginal spasm, pelvic or vaginal pain during sexual intercourse (b) Absence of an identified psychological cause or demonstrable pelvic pathology	625.0, 625.1

Disorders of the menstrual cycle

189	6260	**Menstruation absent, scanty, or rare (amenorrhea, hypomenorrhea, oligomenorrhea)** *excl.* pregnancy (*350,* **V223**) *As defined in the diagnostic title*	626.0, 626.1
190	6262	**Menstruation excessive (hypermenorrhea, menorrhagia), frequent (polymenorrhea), or irregular** *incl.* pubertal bleeding, menometrorrhagia *As defined in the diagnostic title*	626.2–626.4
191	6253	**Menstruation painful (dysmenorrhea) and intermenstrual pain (mittelschmerz)** *Inclusion in this rubric requires:* **A.** *For menstruation painful (dysmenorrhea):* Recurrent episodes of pelvic or abdominal pain during menses, without demonstrable pathology **B.** *For intermenstrual pain (mittelschmerz);* Pelvic, abdominal, or lower back pain occurring at the time of ovulation or approximately midway between menses and lasting less than 24 hours, without demonstrable pathology	625.2, 625.3
192	—	(*Deleted*)	
193	6269	**Intermenstrual bleeding and other disorders of the menstrual cycle** *incl.* metrorrhagia; ovulation bleeding; postcoital bleeding *excl.* postmenopausal bleeding (*187,* **627-**) *As defined in the diagnostic title*	626.5–626.9
194	629-	**Other diseases of the female genitalia** *incl.* Bartholin cyst or abscess; endometriosis; genital tract fistula; leukorrhea; pelvic congestion syndrome; physiological ovarian cyst *excl.* malignant disease (*36,* **180-**) *Inclusion criteria for this rubric are not listed*	616.2–616.9, 617, 619–621, 623, 624, 625.5, 625.8, 625.9, 629

Position no.	ICHPPC code	List of diseases, disorders, and health problems, with inclusion criteria	Comparable ICD-9 codes

Fertility problems

195	**606-**	**Sterility, reduced fertility of male or female**	606, 628

Inclusion in this rubric requires one *of the following:*

(a) Failure to conceive after a 12-month period of normal sexual intercourse without contraception

(b) Evidence of pathology of the generative organs sufficient to reduce fertility

Consider: (338, **V70-***)* If failure to conceive in less than 12 months

Position no.	ICHPPC code	List of diseases, disorders, and health problems, with inclusion criteria	Comparable ICD-9 codes

XI. PREGNANCY, CHILDBIRTH, AND THE PUERPERIUM

196	**633-**	**Ectopic pregnancy** *Inclusion in this rubric requires:* Demonstration of extra-uterine pregnancy by ultrasound, laparoscopy, culdoscopy, or at surgery *Consider:* (*202,* **648-**) Suspected ectopic pregnancy	633
197	**640-**	**Bleeding during pregnancy** *incl.* antepartum hemorrhage—all causes, e.g. placenta previa, abruptio, threatened abortion *As defined in the diagnostic title*	640–641

198	**6466**	**Urinary infection in pregnancy or puerperium**
		incl. asymptomatic bacteriuria
		Inclusion in this rubric requires both *of the following:*
		(a) A diagnosis of urinary infection as defined in the codes (*169,* **5901**), (*170,* **595-**), (*174,* **598-**)
		(b) *One* of the following:
		   (i) A positive diagnosis of pregnancy
		   (ii) Recent termination (within 6 weeks) of pregnancy
			646.5, 646.6

Position no.	ICHPPC code	List of diseases, disorders, and health problems, with inclusion criteria	Comparable ICD-9 codes
199	**642-**	**Toxemia, pre-eclampsia and eclampsia of pregnancy, childbirth, and puerperium** *incl.* hypertension alone, or with one other or more of the triad *excl.* edema, excess weight gain, or albuminuria without hypertension as a complication of pregnancy, childbirth, or in the puerperium (*202,* **648-**) *Inclusion in this rubric requires* both *of the following:* (a) *One* of the following: (i) A positive diagnosis of pregnancy (ii) Recent termination (within 6 weeks) of pregnancy (b) *One* of the following: (i) Elevated blood pressure to a level of at least 90 mm Hg diastolic, at least two readings on two separate occasions, or a rise of at least 15 mm Hg (ii) Elevated blood pressure as defined in (i), one reading, with edema (iii) Elevated blood pressure as defined in (i), one reading, and significant proteinuria (at least 30 mg/100 ml urine) (iv) Convulsions, plus one of the triad of hypertension, edema, and proteinuria	642
200	**636-**	**Abortion, induced, legally or illegally** *incl.* any complications *Inclusion in this rubric requires:* Interruption of an intra-uterine pregnancy by medical or surgical means	635, 636

Position no.	ICHPPC code	List of diseases, disorders, and health problems, with inclusion criteria	Comparable ICD-9 codes
201	**634-**	**Abortion, spontaneous and NOS**	632, 634, 637

634- **Abortion, spontaneous and NOS**
incl. missed and incomplete, and any
complications
excl. threatened abortion (*197*, **640-**)
Inclusion in this rubric requires:
A. *For abortion, spontaneous and NOS, incl.*
incomplete—both *of the following:*
(a) Demonstration of placental or fetal tissue
passed through or present in the vagina,
without a live birth, before 28 weeks'
gestation
(b) Absence of medical or surgical
interventions intended to interrupt
pregnancy
Consider: (*197*, **640-**) Bleeding during
pregnancy; (*202*, **648-**) Premature labor after 28
weeks
B. *For missed abortion*—all *of the following*
before 28 weeks' gestation:
(a) A positive diagnosis of pregnancy
(b) An enlarged, but not enlarging uterus
(c) Death of fetus, as shown by *one* of the
following:
(i) Ultrasound or X-ray evidence
(ii) Two negative pregnancy tests
(iii) Absent fetal movements and heartbeat
Consider: (*253*, **778-**) Fetal death or stillbirth
after 28 weeks

202 **648-** **Other complications of pregnancy (prenatal)**   630, 631, 638, 639,
incl. albuminuria, without hypertension; anemia;   643–645, 646 ex.
edema, without hypertension; emesis and   646.5, (646.6), 647,
hyperemesis; false labor; other conditions   648
complicating pregnancy post-term; premature
labor
excl. coexisting conditions, not complicating
pregnancy; complications of abortion (*200*, **636-**),
(*201*, **634-**)
Inclusion criteria for this rubric are not listed

203 **650-** **Normal delivery**   650
Inclusion in this rubric requires all *of the*
following:
(a) Spontaneous cephalic delivery at term
(b) Absence of fetal manipulation or delivery
with instruments
(c) Absence of abnormality or complications
classifiable elsewhere

Position no.	ICHPPC code	List of diseases, disorders, and health problems, with inclusion criteria	Comparable ICD-9 codes
204	661-	**Complicated delivery and some conditions (diagnosable either during labor and delivery or before) which require special care to avoid complications in pregnancy, labor, or delivery** *incl.* disproportion; elderly primipara; fetal malposition; large-for-dates; multiple pregnancy; old Cesarean section; small-for-dates *Inclusion criteria for this rubric are not listed*	651–669
205	676-	**Mastitis, other disorders of the breast and nipple in the puerperium, and disorders of lactation** *incl.* suppression of lactation *Inclusion in this rubric requires* one *of the following:* (a) A disorder of the nipple or breast which relates to lactation, breast-feeding, or suppression of lactation (b) Suppression of lactation by either medical or mechanical means *Consider:* (*181*, **610-**) Chronic cystic disease of breast; (*182*, **611-**) Other breast disorders	675–676
206	670-	**Other complications of puerperium (postnatal)** *incl.* infection of genital tract; postoperative complications of obstetrical surgery *excl.* anemia (*202*, **648-**); toxemia syndromes (*199*, **642**); urinary infection (*198*, **6466**) *Inclusion criteria for this rubric are not listed*	pt. 646.6, 670–674

Position no.	ICHPPC code	List of diseases, disorders, and health problems, with inclusion criteria	Comparable ICD-9 codes

XII. DISEASES OF THE SKIN AND SUBCUTANEOUS TISSUE

207 **680-** **Boil, carbuncle, cellulitis, abscess** 680–682
incl. finger, toe, with or without lymphangitis; paronychia
excl. inside of nose (*146*, **4781**); perianal (*162*, **565-**); male external genitalia (*180*, **607-**); female external genitalia (*194*, **629-**); lymphadenitis (*209*, **683-**); wound infection (*333*, **959-**)
Inclusion in this rubric requires:
A. *For boil, carbuncle, abscess:*
Localized, tender swelling containing pus in a region not excluded in the diagnostic title
B. *For cellulitis:*
Inflammatory lesion of skin involving subcutaneous tissue which has increased warmth, redness, and indistinct borders in a region not excluded in the diagnostic title

208 — (*Deleted*)

209 **683-** **Lymphadenitis, acute** 683
incl. abscess of lymph node
excl. chronic lymphadenitis (*63*, **2891**); enlarged lymph node NOS (*266*, **7856**); mesenteric lymphadenitis (*63*, **2891**)
Inclusion in this rubric requires:
One or more enlarged, tender or painful lymph nodes in the same anatomical location, which are of recent onset (less than 6 weeks) and where the primary source of infection is unknown

210 **684-** **Impetigo** 684
incl. impetigo secondary to other dermatoses
Inclusion in this rubric requires:
One or more inflammatory lesions, not resulting from injury, with a thick honey-coloured crust
Consider: (*333*, **959-**) if secondary to injury

211 **685-** **Pilonidal cyst, fistula, pyoderma, pyogenic granuloma, infected sinus, ecthyma and other infections of the skin and subcutaneous tissue** 685, 686
Inclusion criteria for this rubric are not listed

Position no.	ICHPPC code	List of diseases, disorders, and health problems, with inclusion criteria	Comparable ICD-9 codes
212	690-	**Seborrheic dermatitis and other erythematosquamous dermatoses** *incl.* dandruff	690

Inclusion criteria are not listed for part of this rubric
For optional hierarchy, inclusion in this rubric requires:
A. *For dandruff:*
Flaking and scaling of the skin of the scalp or eyebrow not attributable to other skin disease
B. *For other seborrheic dermatitis:*
One or more areas of chronic erythema with greasy scales, showing a predilection for these areas of the skin: scalp, face, neck, upper trunk, axilla, groin, anogenital region
C. *For other erythematosquamous dermatoses—inclusion criteria for this part of the rubric are not listed*
Consider: (277, **709-***)* Seborrheic warts, hyperkeratoses; *(292,* **7821***)* Rash NOS

| 213 | 6918 | **Atopic dermatitis or eczema** *incl.* infantile eczema and flexural dermatitis *excl.* diaper rash (*215,* **6910**) | 691.8 |

Inclusion in this rubric requires:
A pruritic skin lesion with erythema, vesiculation, weeping, crusting, peeling, or lichenification and *three* of the following:
(a) Predilection for flexural areas (under the age of 2 predilection for face, scalp, extensor aspects of limbs, trunk, diaper area)
(b) Onset in infancy
(c) Chronic relapsing course
(d) Associated with asthma, allergic rhinitis, or allergic conjunctivitis
(e) Personal or family history of atopy

Position no.	ICHPPC code	List of diseases, disorders, and health problems, with inclusion criteria	Comparable ICD-9 codes
214	692-	**Contact dermatitis and other eczema or dermatitis** *incl.* dermatitis NOS; due to cold or hot weather; due to drugs taken internally or externally; eczema NOS; sunburn *excl.* allergy NOS, allergic reaction NOS (*378*, **9950**); contact and other dermatitis of the eyelid (*93*, **3730**); diaper rash (*215*, **6910**); rash NOS (*292*, **7821**) *Inclusion in this rubric requires:* **A.** *For contact dermatitis*—both *of the following:* (a) Identification of an etiological contact agent (b) Dermatitis in the area of contact **B.** *For other eczema or dermatitis:* A pruritic skin lesion with erythema, vesiculation, weeping, crusting, peeling, or lichenification *Consider:* (*218*, **698-**) Pruritus, neurodermatitis	692, 693
215	6910	**Diaper rash (napkin rash)** *Inclusion in this rubric requires* both *of the following:* (a) Dermatitis, primarily of the diaper area, in infants (b) Absence of inclusion criteria required for other rubrics in this section	691.0
216	6963	**Pityriasis rosea** *Inclusion in this rubric requires:* A rash, with *three* of the following: (i) An initial 'herald patch' (ii) Pink, slightly scaly, lesions (iii) Predominantly oval lesions which follow skin cleavage lines (iv) Lesions primarily on trunk, neck, and upper aspects of extremities	696.3
217	6961	**Psoriasis, with or without arthropathy** *Inclusion in this rubric requires* one *of the following:* (a) Characteristic histological appearance (b) Typical morphological appearance of the skin (thick micaceous scaly lesions, with punctate bleeding after scraping away of scales, primarily confined to the elbows, knees, scalp, and sacrum) (c) *Two* of the following, when rash is atypical: (i) Pitted nails (ii) Family history of psoriasis (iii) Chronic course (iv) Arthropathy	696.0, 696.1

Position no.	ICHPPC code	List of diseases, disorders, and health problems, with inclusion criteria	Comparable ICD-9 codes
218	698-	**Pruritus and related conditions** *incl.* anogenital pruritus; dermatitis factitia; itch NOS; lichen simplex chronicus; neurodermatitis *excl.* rash NOS (*292*, **7821**) *Inclusion criteria for this rubric are not listed*	698
219	700-	**Corns, callosities** *Inclusion in this rubric requires:* Thickened hyperkeratotic skin in *one* of the following situations: (i) Over a bony prominence (natural or pathological) (ii) In an area of skin subjected to unusual friction or pressure	700
220	7062	**Sebaceous cyst** *incl.* inclusion dermoid *Inclusion in this rubric requires:* A localized cystic mass situated in the epidermis, but attached to the dermis	706.2
221	703-	**Ingrowing toenail, onychogryphosis, and other diseases of the nail** *Inclusion criteria for this rubric are not listed*	703
222	704-	**Alopecia, folliculitis, and other diseases of the hair** *incl.* sycosis barbae *Inclusion criteria for this rubric are not listed*	704
223	705-	**Pompholyx, other diseases of sweat glands** *incl.* dyshidrosis; heat rash; miliaria; prickly heat; sweat rash *excl.* hyperhidrosis (*290*, **7808**) *Inclusion criteria for this rubric are not listed*	705
224	7061	**Acne** *excl.* acne rosacea (*227*, **709-**) *Inclusion in this rubric requires* all *of the following:* (a) Multiple lesions (which may be any of the following: comedones, papules, pustules, abscesses, cysts, scars, pitting) (b) Distribution on the face and upper thorax and back (c) Onset in 2nd and 3rd decades of life or in association with exposure to industrial irritants or medications (hormones, halides) *Consider:* (*207*, **680-**) if few lesions or atypical distribution	706.0, 706.1

Position no.	ICHPPC code	List of diseases, disorders, and health problems, with inclusion criteria	Comparable ICD-9 codes
225	707-	**Chronic ulcer of skin** *incl.* bedsore; pressure sore *excl.* varicose ulcer (*129*, **454-**) *As defined in the diagnostic title*	707
226	708-	**Urticaria** *excl.* angioedema, allergic edema (*378*, **9950**); drug allergy (*377*, **9952**); edema NOS (*265*, **7823**) *Inclusion in this rubric requires:* Circumscribed raised areas of edema limited to superficial portion of the dermis	708
227	709-	**Other disease of the skin and subcutaneous tissue** *incl.* acne rosacea; erythema multiforme; erythema nodosum; erythema NOS; granuloma; ichthyosis; intertrigo; keloid; lichen planus; hyperkeratosis; localized lupus erythematosus; seborrheic or senile warts; solar keratosis; striae atrophicae; vitiligo *excl.* warts (*19*, **0781**); malignant skin lesions (*34*, **173-**); mole (*41*, **216-**); pigmented nevus (*41*, **216-**) *Inclusion criteria for this rubric are not listed*	694, 695, 696.2, 696.4–696.8, 697, 701, 702, 706.3, 706.9, 709

Position no.	ICHPPC code	List of diseases, disorders, and health problems, with inclusion criteria	Comparable ICD-9 codes

XIII. DISEASES OF THE MUSCULOSKELETAL SYSTEM AND CONNECTIVE TISSUE ARTHRITIS AND ARTHROSIS

228	**714-**	**Rheumatoid arthritis and allied conditions**	714, 720.0

incl. ankylosing spondylitis
excl. psoriatic arthropathy (*217*, **6961**)
Inclusion in this rubric requires:
A. *For rheumatoid arthritis—all of the following:*
(a) Presence or history of an episode of joint pain involving three or more limb joints which occur in groups (e.g. PIPs or MCPs on one side count only as a single joint)
(b) Swelling, subluxation, or ankylosis of at least three limb joints including one hand, wrist, or foot with symmetry of at least one joint pair (Joints *excluded* are hips, DIPs, fifth PIPs, first CMCs and first MTPs)
(c) X-ray features of grade 2, 3, or more of erosive arthritis in the hands, wrists, or feet
(d) Positive serological reaction for rheumatoid factor
B. *For ankylosing spondylitis:*
Characteristic radiological appearance
Consider: (*288*, **7194**) Pain in joint; (*289*, **7190**) Swelling of joint; (*231*, **725-**) Arthritis NYD or NOS

229	**715-**	**Osteoarthrosis (osteoarthritis) and allied conditions**	715

excl. of spine (*237*, **721-**)
Inclusion in this rubric requires one *of the following:*
(a) Characteristic radiological appearance
(b) Heberden's nodes
(c) Joint disorder of at least 3 months' duration, with no constitutional symptoms and *three* of the following:
(i) Irregular swelling
(ii) Crepitation
(iii) Stiffness or limitation of movement
(iv) Normal ESR, rheumatoid tests, and uric acid
(v) Over 40 years of age
Consider: (*288*, **7194**) Pain in joint; (*289*, **7190**) Swelling of joint; (*231*, **725-**) Arthritis NYD or NOS

Position no.	ICHPPC code	List of diseases, disorders, and health problems, with inclusion criteria	Comparable ICD-9 codes
230	**7161**	**Traumatic arthropathy (arthritis)** *excl.* effusion (*289*, **7190**); internal derangement of knee—acute (*312*, **836-**), chronic (*244*, **717-**) *Inclusion in this rubric requires:* Joint disorder beginning with trauma and persisting for more than three months in the absence of other causes of joint pain *Consider:* (*288*, **7194**) Pain in joint; (*289*, **7190**) Swelling of joint; (*231*, **725-**) Arthritis NYD or NOS	716.1
(*288*)	**7194**	**Pain in joint, arthralgia, stiffness in joint** *Inclusion in this rubric requires:* The above symptom(s), but without additional criteria needed for inclusion in other rubrics	719.4, 719.5
(*289*)	**7190**	**Swelling of joint, effusion of joint** with or without pain *Inclusion in this rubric requires:* The above symptom(s), but without additional criteria needed for inclusion in other rubrics	719.0
231	**725-**	**Other types of arthritis and diffuse connective tissue disorders** *incl.* arthritis secondary to other diseases; arthritis NYD or NOS; chondrocalcinoses, other; dermatomyositis; palindromic rheumatism; polymyalgia rheumatica; pyogenic arthritis; scleroderma (progressive); systemic lupus erythematosus; villonodular synovitis *Inclusion criteria for this rubric are not listed*	710–713, 716 ex. 716.1, 719.2, 719.3, 725

Non-articular rheumatism

232	**7260**	**The shoulder syndromes** *incl.* bursitis of shoulder; frozen shoulder; rotator cuff syndrome; synovitis of shoulder; tendinitis around shoulder *Inclusion in this rubric requires:* Shoulder pain, with *one* of the following: (a) Limitation of movement (b) Local tenderness (c) Periarticular calcification on radiography	726.0–726.2

Position no.	ICHPPC code	List of diseases, disorders, and health problems, with inclusion criteria	Comparable ICD-9 codes
233	**7263**	**Other bursitis, tendinitis, tenosynovitis, synovitis and peripheral enthesopathy** *incl.* bone spur; calcified tendon; peritendinitis; synovial cyst; tennis elbow *excl.* of shoulder (*232*, **7260**); of spine (*238*, **7242**), (*239*, **7244**); ganglion (*241*, **7274**); bunion (*245*, **736-**) *Inclusion criteria for this rubric are not listed*	726.3–726.9, 727 (ex. 727.1, 727.4)
234	**728-**	**Other non-articular rheumatism and disorders of muscle, ligament, and fascia** *incl.* Dupuytren's contracture; fasciitis; fibrositis; foreign-body granuloma; muscle pain; myalgia; myositis; panniculitis *excl.* epidemic myositis (Bornholm's disease) (*31*, **136-**); sprains and strains, Section XVII *Inclusion criteria for this rubric are not listed*	728, 729 (ex. 729.5, 729.8)
(*286*)	**7295**	**Pain and other symptoms referrable to limbs** *incl.* 'growing pains' in a child; leg cramps *excl.* pain in spine (*238*, **7242**); (*239*, **7244**); restless legs syndrome (*91*, **355-**) *Inclusion in this rubric requires:* The above symptom(s), but without additional criteria needed for inclusion in other rubrics	729.4, 729.8

Syndromes related to the vertebral column

235	**723-**	**Syndromes related to the cervical spine** *incl.* cervical disc lesion; cervicalgia; cervicobrachial syndrome; radicular syndrome of upper limbs; torticollis *excl.* psychogenic tension headache (*76*, **3078**); osteoarthritis of spine (*237*, **721-**); cervical strain (*319*, **8470**) *Inclusion criteria for this rubric are not listed*	722.0, 722.4, 723
236	—	(*Deleted*)	
237	**721-**	**Osteoarthritis of spine** (any region) *incl.* spondylosis *Inclusion in this rubric requires:* Characteristic radiological appearance *Consider:* (*238*, **7242**) if no positive X-ray findings	721

Position no.	ICHPPC code	List of diseases, disorders, and health problems, with inclusion criteria	Comparable ICD-9 codes
238	**7242**	**Back pain (lumbar, thoracic, or sacroiliac) without radiating symptoms** *incl.* backache NOS; coccydynia; lumbago; lumbalgia *excl.* psychogenic backache (*76*, **3078**); spondylolisthesis (*252*, **758-**); recent back strain (*320*, **8478**) *As defined in the diagnostic title*	720.1–720.9, 724.1, 724.2, 724.5–724.9
239	**7244**	**Back pain (lumbar or thoracic) with radiating symptoms** *incl.* prolapsed or degenerated disc; sciatica *excl.* spondylolisthesis (*252*, **758-**); recent back strain (*320*, **8478**) *Inclusion in this rubric requires one of the following:* (a) Demonstration of a prolapsed lumbar or thoracic disc by appropriate radiological technique, or at surgery (b) Pain in the lumbar or thoracic region of the spine, accompanied by pain radiating to, or a neurological deficit of, an appropriate area (c) Sciatica, pain radiating down the back of the leg, aggravated by coughing, movement, or posture	722.1, 722.5, 724.3, 724.4
240	**737-**	**Acquired deformities of spine** *incl.* curvature NOS; kyphoscoliosis; kyphosis; lordosis; scoliosis *excl.* ankylosing spondylitis (*228*, **714-**); congenital deformities (*252*, **758-**); spondylolisthesis (*252*, **758-**) *Inclusion criteria for this rubric are not listed*	737

Other musculoskeletal and connective tissue disorders

241	**7274**	**Ganglion** of joint (capsule) and tendon (sheath) *Inclusion in this rubric requires:* Firm cystic swelling, not attached to skin, but related to tendon or joint	727.4

Position no.	ICHPPC code	List of diseases, disorders, and health problems, with inclusion criteria	Comparable ICD-9 codes
242	**732-**	**Osgood–Schlatter's disease, other osteochondroses and osteochondropathies** *incl.* Legg–Calve–Perthes disease; osteochondritis dissecans; Scheuermann's disease; slipped femoral epiphysis *Inclusion criteria are not listed for part of this rubric* *For optional hierarchy, inclusion in this rubric requires:* **A.** *For Osgood–Schlatter's disease—one of the following:* (a) Painful, tender, swollen, non-traumatic tibial tubercle in a young person, not due to acute trauma (b) Characteristic radiological appearance **B.** *For osteochondroses and osteochondropathies—inclusion criteria for this part of the rubric are not given*	732
243	**7330**	**Osteoporosis** *Inclusion in this rubric requires:* Characteristic radiological appearance *Note:* Double code if etiology identified	733.0
244	**717-**	**Chronic internal derangement of knee** *incl.* chondromalacia patella; longstanding meniscus tear; loose body in knee *excl.* acute current injury (*312*, **836-**); recurrent dislocation (*246*, **739-**); *Inclusion in this rubric requires* one *of the following:* (a) A history of at least one previous similar episode (b) A history of current episode lasting for at least one month	717
245	**736-**	**Acquired deformities of limbs** *incl.* bunion; genu valgum-varum; hallux valgus-varus-rigidus; mallet finger; pes planus (flatfoot) *excl.* congenital deformities and anomalies (*248*, **754-**), (*252*, **758-**) *Inclusion criteria for this rubric are not listed*	727.1, 734–736

Position no.	ICHPPC code	List of diseases, disorders, and health problems, with inclusion criteria	Comparable ICD-9 codes
246	**739-**	**Other diseases of the musculoskeletal system and connective tissue** *incl.* arthrodesis; costochondritis; joint mice (excl. knee); malunion or non-union of fracture; osteomyelitis; Paget's disease of bone; pathological fracture NOS; post-surgical back pain; recurrent dislocation; weakness in limb muscle or joint NOS *excl.* curvature of spine (*240,* **737-**); late effects of polio (*8,* **045-**); trigger finger (*233,* **7263**); curvature of spine (*240,* **737-**) *Inclusion criteria for this rubric are not listed*	718, 719.1, 719.6–719.9, 722.2, 722.3, 722.6–722.9, 724.0, 730, 731, 733 ex. 733.0, 738, 739

Position no.	ICHPPC code	List of diseases, disorders, and health problems, with inclusion criteria	Comparable ICD-9 codes

XIV. CONGENITAL ANOMALIES

247	**746-**	**Congenital anomalies of the heart and circulatory system** *Inclusion criteria for this rubric are not listed*	745–747
248	**754-**	**Certain congenital anomalies of lower limb** *incl.* bowing of long bones of leg; clubfoot (all types); congenital dislocation of hip; genu recurvatum; other congenital deformities of the foot *excl.* pes planus (acquired) (*245*, **736-**) *Inclusion in this rubric requires:* Evidence that the condition began in the first two years of life	754.3–754.7
249	**7525**	**Undescended testicle** *Inclusion in this rubric requires* both *of the following:* (a) The testicle has never been observed in the scrotum (b) The testicle cannot be manipulated into the scrotum	752.5
250	—	(*Deleted*)	
251	**7436**	**Blocked tear duct, agenesis of the lacrimal punctum** *Inclusion in this rubric requires:* Overflow of tears without crying, beginning before the age of three months	pt. 743.6
252	**758-**	**Other congenital anomalies** *incl.* birthmarks (excl. hemangioma); cleft lip and palate; congenital polycystic kidneys; Darwin's tubercle; Down's syndrome; Meckel's diverticulum; spina bifida; spondylolisthesis; supernumerary nipples; tongue-tie; webbed fingers *excl.* hemangioma, lymphangioma (*44*, **228-**); congenital xanthoma (*56*, **272-**); congenital metabolic disorders (e.g. cystic fibrosis) (Section III) *Inclusion criteria for this rubric are not listed*	740–742, 743 (ex. pt. 743.6) 744, 748–751, 752 (ex. 752.5) 753, 754 (ex. 754.3–754.7), 755–759

Position no.	ICHPPC code	List of diseases, disorders, and health problems, with inclusion criteria	Comparable ICD-9 codes

XV. CERTAIN CONDITIONS ORIGINATING IN THE PERINATAL PERIOD

| *253* | 778- | **All perinatal morbidity and mortality conditions** | 760–779 |

incl. diarrhea of newborn; dysmature or postmature newborn; factors in labor and delivery as they affect the fetus or newborn; feeding problems in the neonatal period; hemolytic disease of newborn; maternal conditions as they affect the fetus or newborn; one of multiple birth; physiological jaundice; pneumonia of the newborn; respiratory distress syndrome; umbilical sepsis

excl. congenital conditions (Section XIV); failure to thrive NOS (*294*, **7834**)

Inclusion criteria for this rubric are not listed

Position no.	ICHPPC code	List of diseases, disorders, and health problems, with inclusion criteria	Comparable ICD-9 codes

XVI. SYMPTOMS, SIGNS, AND ILL-DEFINED CONDITIONS

Note: The term 'symptom' includes both symptoms and signs, as normally understood.

Inclusion in each of the rubrics in this section requires that the symptom(s) indicated represent the most specific diagnosis it is possible to make at the time of the encounter; if the symptom(s) can confidently be attributed to a more specific diagnosis, the rubric in this section should not be used.

If the symptom or sign is considered a normal variant, code (*338,* **V70-**), unless a variant of the aging process, in which case code (*297,* **797-**). Except where indicated, these symptoms can be accepted on the subjective assessment of the patient, without requiring objective confirmation by the health care provider.

Position no.	ICHPPC code	List of diseases, disorders, and health problems, with inclusion criteria	Comparable ICD-9 codes

XVI. SYMPTOMS, SIGNS, AND ILL-DEFINED CONDITIONS

Central nervous system and peripheral nerves

254   **7803**   **Convulsions**   780.3
incl. febrile convulsions
excl. convulsions in newborn (*253*, **778-**)
Inclusion in this rubric requires:
The above symptom(s), but without additional
criteria needed for inclusion in other rubrics

255   **7810**   **Abnormal involuntary movement**   781.0
incl. fasciculation; tremor spasms
excl. tic, habit spasm (*86*, **316-**); restless legs
syndrome (*91*, **355-**); Sydenham's chorea
(*108*, **390**)
Inclusion in this rubric requires:
The above symptom(s), but without additional
criteria needed for inclusion in other rubrics

256   **7804**   **Dizziness, giddiness**   780.4
excl. specific vertiginous syndromes (*104*, **386-**)
Inclusion in this rubric requires:
The above symptom(s), but without additional
criteria needed for inclusion in other rubrics
Consider: (*264*, **7802**) Syncope, blackout

257   **7845**   **Disturbance of speech**   784.3–784.5
incl. hoarseness
excl. stammering, stuttering (*86*, **316-**)
Inclusion in this rubric requires:
The above symptom(s), but without additional
criteria needed for inclusion in other rubrics

258   **7840**   **Headache**   784.0
incl. pain in head or face NOS
excl. tension headache (*76*, **3078**); migraine (*90*,
346-); atypical facial neuralgia (*91*, **355-**)
Inclusion in this rubric requires:
The above symptom(s), but without additional
criteria needed for inclusion in other rubrics

259   **7820**   **Disturbance of sensation, paresthesias**   782.0
excl. restless legs syndrome (*91*, **355-**)
Inclusion in this rubric requires:
The above symptom(s), but without additional
criteria needed for inclusion in other rubrics

260   —   (*Deleted*)

261   —   (*Deleted*)

Position no.	ICHPPC code	List of diseases, disorders, and health problems, with inclusion criteria	Comparable ICD-9 codes

Cardiovascular and lymphatic systems

262	**7865**	**Chest pain** *incl.* painful respiration; pleuritic pain; pleurodynia; precordial pain *Inclusion in this rubric requires:* The above symptom(s), but without additional criteria needed for inclusion in other rubrics	786.5
263	**7851**	**Palpitation (aware of heartbeat)** *Inclusion in this rubric requires:* The above symptom(s), but without additional criteria needed for inclusion in other rubrics *Consider:* (*300*, **7889**) Tachycardia NOS	785.1
264	**7802**	**Syncope, faint, blackout** *Inclusion in this rubric requires:* The above symptom(s), but without additional criteria needed for inclusion in other rubrics *Consider:* (*256*, **7804**) Giddiness, dizziness	780.2
(116)	**7852**	**Heart murmur NEC or NYD;** functional, innocent *Inclusion in this rubric requires:* The above symptom(s), but without additional criteria needed for inclusion in other rubrics	785.2, pt. 785.9
265	**7823**	**Edema—localized or dependent** *excl.* fluid retention (*57*, **279**); in pregnancy (*199*, **642-**), (*202*, **648-**); allergic (*378*, **9950**) *Inclusion in this rubric requires:* The above symptom(s), but without additional criteria needed for inclusion in other rubrics *Note:* Requires objective verification *Consider:* (*296*, **7822**) Localized swelling	782.3
266	**7856**	**Enlarged lymph nodes, not infected** *incl.* lymphadenopathy *excl.* lymphadenitis—acute (*209*, **683-**)—chronic (*63*, **2891**) *Inclusion in this rubric requires:* The above symptom(s), but without additional criteria needed for inclusion in other rubrics *Note:* Requires objective verification	785.6

Position no.	ICHPPC code	List of diseases, disorders, and health problems, with inclusion criteria	Comparable ICD-9 codes

Respiratory system

267	**7847**	**Epistaxis** *Inclusion in this rubric requires:* The above symptom, but without additional criteria needed for inclusion in other rubrics	784.7
268	**7863**	**Hemoptysis** *Inclusion in this rubric requires:* The above symptom, but without additional criteria needed for inclusion in other rubrics	786.3
269	**7860**	**Dyspnea** *incl.* orthopnea; stridor; tachypnea; wheezing *excl.* hyperventilation of psychogenic origin (*71,* **3001**); respiratory distress of newborn (*253,* **778-**); respiratory failure (*300,* **7889**) *Inclusion in this rubric requires:* The above symptom(s), but without additional criteria needed for inclusion in other rubrics	786.0, 786.1
270	**7862**	**Cough** *Inclusion in this rubric requires:* The above symptom, but without additional criteria needed for inclusion in other rubrics	786.2
271	—	(*Deleted*)	
272	—	(*Deleted*)	

Gastro-intestinal system and abdomen

273	**7830**	**Anorexia** *Inclusion in this rubric requires:* The above symptom, but without additional criteria needed for inclusion in other rubrics	783.0
274	**7870**	**Nausea and/or vomiting** *excl.* of newborn (*253,* **778-**); or pregnancy (*202,* **648-**) *Inclusion in this rubric requires:* The above symptom, but without additional criteria needed for inclusion in other rubrics	787.0
275	**7871**	**Heartburn** *Inclusion in this rubric requires* The above symptom, but without additional criteria needed for inclusion in other rubrics *Consider:* (*153,* **536-**) Indigestion NOS	787.1
276	—	(*Deleted*)	

Position no.	ICHPPC code	List of diseases, disorders, and health problems, with inclusion criteria	Comparable ICD-9 codes
277	7891	**Hepatomegaly and/or splenomegaly** *Inclusion in this rubric requires:* The above symptom(s), but without additional criteria needed for inclusion in other rubrics *Note:* Requires objective verification	789.1, 789.2
278	7873	**Gas problems (wind)** *incl.* bloating; eructation; flatulence; gas pains in the adult; passage of excess gas per rectum *Inclusion in this rubric requires:* The above symptom(s), but without additional criteria needed for inclusion in other rubrics	787.3
279	7890	**Abdominal pain** *incl.* infantile colic *Inclusion in this rubric requires:* The above symptom(s), but without additional criteria needed for inclusion in other rubrics *Consider:* (*153*, **536-**) Indigestion NOS	789.0

Genito-urinary system

280	7881	**Dysuria** *Inclusion in this rubric requires:* The above symptom, but without additional criteria needed for inclusion in other rubrics *Consider:* (*283*, **7884**) Frequency of urination	788.1
281	7883	**Enuresis, bedwetting, urinary incontinence** *excl.* clearly of psychogenic origin (*86*, **316-**); stress incontinence NOS (*186*, **618-**) *Inclusion in this rubric requires:* The above symptom(s), but without additional criteria needed for inclusion in other rubrics	788.3
282	—	(*Deleted*)	
283	7884	**Frequency of urination** *incl.* nocturia; polyuria *Inclusion in this rubric requires:* The above symptom(s), but without additional criteria needed for inclusion in other rubrics	788.4
284	—	(*Deleted*)	
285	—	(*Deleted*)	
286	7295	(See after position number 234)	
287	—	(*Deleted*)	
288	7194	(See after position number 230)	
289	7190	(See after position numbers 230, 288)	

Position no.	ICHPPC code	List of diseases, disorders, and health problems, with inclusion criteria	Comparable ICD-9 codes

General signs and symptoms

290	7808	**Excessive sweating, hyperhidrosis** *Inclusion in this rubric requires:* The above symptom(s), but without additional criteria needed for inclusion in other rubrics	780.8
291	7806	**Fever of undetermined cause (pyrexia of unknown origin), hyperpyrexia** *Inclusion in this rubric requires:* The above symptom(s), but without additional criteria needed for inclusion in other rubrics	780.6
292	7821	**Rash and other non-specific skin eruptions** *excl.* rash with pyrexia NOS (*14*, **057-**) *Inclusion in this rubric requires:* The above symptom(s), but without additional criteria needed for inclusion in other rubrics	782.1
293	7832	**Weight loss, cachexia** *Inclusion in this rubric requires:* An involuntary weight loss of at least 10% of body weight *Consider:* (*338*, **V70-**) for minimal weight loss of less than 10%	783.2, 799.4
294	7834	**Lack of expected physiological development, failure to thrive** *excl.* learning disorder (*74*, **315-**); mental retardation (*85*, **317-**) *Inclusion in this rubric requires:* The above symptom(s), but without additional criteria needed for inclusion in other rubrics	783.4
(*53*)	7833	**Feeding problem: baby or elderly** *excl.* feeding problem in neonatal period (*253*, **778-**) *Inclusion in this rubric requires:* The above symptom(s), but without additional criteria needed for inclusion in other rubrics	783.3
295	7807	**Malaise, debility, fatigue, tiredness** *incl.* postviral syndromes *excl.* neurasthenia (*73*, **3009**) *Inclusion in this rubric requires:* The above symptom(s), but without additional criteria needed for inclusion in other rubrics	780.7, 799.3

Position no.	ICHPPC code	List of diseases, disorders, and health problems, with inclusion criteria	Comparable ICD-9 codes
296	7822	**Mass, lump, or localized swelling in abdomen, pelvis, chest, head and neck, skin and subcutaneous tissues** *excl.* breast (*182*, **611-**); enlarged lymph node (*266*, **7856**); swelling of joint (*289*, **7190**) *Inclusion in this rubric requires:* The above symptom(s), but without additional criteria needed for inclusion in other rubrics	782.2, 784.2, 786.6, 789.3
297	797-	**Senility, senescence** *excl.* senile dementia (*66*, **294-**) *Inclusion in this rubric requires:* Problems related to aging, but without additional criteria needed for inclusion in other rubrics	797

Investigations with unexplained abnormal results

298	791-	**Other abnormal urine test finding** *incl.* glucosuria; proteinuria *excl.* metabolic disorders involving amino acids and certain carbohydrates (*57*, **279-**); orthostatic albuminuria (*173*, **5936**) *Inclusion in this rubric requires:* The above symptom(s), but without additional criteria needed for inclusion in other rubrics *Note:* Requires objective verification	791
(*375*)	7900	**Other hematological abnormalities** *incl.* red cell abnormalities; raised ESR *excl.* anemia(s) (*58*, **280-** to *61*, **285-**); anemia in pregnancy (*202*, **648-**); polycythemia rubra vera (*46*, **239-**) *Inclusion in this rubric requires:* The above symptom(s), but without additional criteria needed for inclusion in other rubrics *Note:* Requires objective verification	790.0, 790.1
(*51*)	7902	**Abnormal unexplained blood test** *incl.* bacteremia; abnormal glucose tolerance test; hyperglycemia; hyperuricemia; multiphasic biochemical screening (SMA) abnormality *excl.* disorders of fluids, electrolytes, acid–base balance (*57*, **279-**); lipids (*56*, **272-**); hypoglycemia (*57*, **279-**); renal failure, uremia (*174*, **598-**) *Inclusion in this rubric requires:* The above symptom(s), but without additional criteria needed for inclusion in other rubrics *Note:* Requires objective verification	250.9

Position no.	ICHPPC code	List of diseases, disorders, and health problems, with inclusion criteria	Comparable ICD-9 codes
(376)	**7950**	**Non-specific abnormal pap smear** *excl.* carcinoma *in situ* of cervix (*36*, **180-**); cervicitis, cervical dysplasia (*184*, **622-**) *Inclusion in this rubric requires:* The above symptom, but without additional criteria needed for inclusion in other rubrics *Note:* Requires objective verification	795.0
(119)	**7962**	**Elevated blood-pressure without a diagnosis of hypertension (hyperpiesia, hyperpiesis)** *Inclusion in this rubric requires:* The above symptom, but without additional criteria needed for inclusion in other rubrics *Note:* Requires objective verification	796.2
299	**793-**	**Other investigations with unexplained abnormal results** *incl.* ECG; function studies; histology, serology; ultrasound; X-rays *Inclusion in this rubric requires:* The above symptom(s), but without additional criteria needed for inclusion in other rubrics *Note:* Requires objective verification	792–794, 795 ex. 795.0, 796 ex. 796.2

All other signs, symptoms and ill-defined conditions

300	**7889**	**All other signs, symptoms and ill-defined conditions** *incl.* any poorly understood condition which is under observation NEC; abnormal gait; ascites; cyanosis; death of unknown or undetermined origin; fecal incontinence; gangrene; halitosis; hiccough; jaundice; pallor; renal colic; respiratory failure; tachycardia NOS; urethral discharge NOS; urine retention *excl.* fluid and electrolyte disturbance (*57*, **279-**); stridor (*269*, **7860**); normal variant (*338*, **V70-**) *Inclusion in this rubric requires:* The above symptom(s), but without additional criteria needed for inclusion in other rubrics	780.0, 780.1, 780.5, 780.9, 781 ex. 781.0, 782.4–782.9, 783.1, 783.5–783.9, 784.1, 784.6, 784.8, 784.9, 785.0, 785.3–785.5, pt. 785.9, 786.4, 786.7–786.9, 787.2, 787.4–787.9, 788.0, 788.2, 788.5–788.9, 789.4–789.9, 798, 799 (ex. 799.3, 799.4)

Position no.	ICHPPC code	List of diseases, disorders, and health problems, with inclusion criteria	Comparable ICD-9 codes

XVII. ACCIDENTS, INJURY, POISONING, AND VIOLENCE

Fractures excl. malunion, non-union (*246,* **739-**)

301	802-	**Skull and facial bones**	800–804

Inclusion in this rubric requires both *of the following:*
(a) Trauma to the bone
(b) *One* of the following:
   (i) X-ray evidence of a fracture
   (ii) Palpable displacement of the bone surface
Consider: (*322,* **850-**) Head injury;
(*327,* **929-**) Bruise, contusion

302	805-	**Vertebral column, with or without cord lesion**	805–806

Inclusion in this rubric requires both *of the following:*
(a) Trauma to the bone
(b) X-ray evidence of a fracture
Consider: (*333,* **959-**) if no X-ray

303	807-	**Ribs**	807.0, 807.1

Inclusion in this rubric requires both *of the following:*
(a) Trauma to the bone
(b) *One* of the following:
   (i) X-ray evidence of a fracture
   (ii) Pain (worse with breathing) with localized tenderness or crepitus involving the bone
Consider: (*327,* **929-**) Bruise, contusion

304	810-	**Clavicle**	810

Inclusion in this rubric requires both *of the following:*
(a) Trauma to the bone
(b) *One* of the following:
   (i) X-ray evidence of a fracture
   (ii) Visible or palpable deformity or crepitus involving the bone
Consider: (*327,* **929-**) Bruise, contusion

Position no.	ICHPPC code	List of diseases, disorders, and health problems, with inclusion criteria	Comparable ICD-9 codes

305	**812-**	**Humerus**
		 Inclusion in this rubric requires both *of the following:*
		 (a) Trauma to the bone
		 (b) *One* of the following:
		    (i) X-ray evidence of a fracture
		    (ii) Visible or palpable deformity or crepitus involving the bone
		 Consider: (*327,* **929-**) Bruise, contusion
			812

306	**813-**	**Radius, ulna**
		 incl. Colles' fracture
		 Inclusion in this rubric requires both *of the following:*
		 (a) Trauma to the bone
		 (b) *One* of the following
		    (i) X-ray evidence of a fracture
		    (ii) Visible or palpable deformity or crepitus involving the bone
		 Consider: (*327,* **929-**) Bruise, contusion
			813

307	**814-**	**Carpal, metacarpal, tarsal, metatarsal bones**
		 Inclusion in this rubric requires both *of the following:*
		 (a) Trauma to the bone
		 (b) *One* of the following:
		    (i) X-ray evidence of a fracture
		    (ii) Visible or palpable deformity or crepitus involving the bone
		 Consider: (*327,* **929-**) Bruise, contusion
			814, 815, 825

308-	**816-**	**Phalanges of foot or hand**
		 Inclusion in this rubric requires both *of the following:*
		 (a) Trauma to the bone
		 (b) *One* of the following:
		    (i) X-ray evidence of a fracture
		    (ii) Visible or palpable deformity or crepitus involving the bone
		 Consider: (*327,* **929-**) Bruise, contusion
			816, 826

309	**820-**	**Femur**
		 Inclusion in this rubric requires both *of the following:*
		 (a) Trauma to the bone
		 (b) *One* of the following:
		    (i) X-ray evidence of a fracture
		    (ii) Visible or palpable deformity or crepitus involving the bone
		 Consider: (*327,* **929-**) Bruise, contusion
			820, 821

Position no.	ICHPPC code	List of diseases, disorders, and health problems, with inclusion criteria	Comparable ICD-9 codes
310	823-	**Tibia, fibula** *incl.* Pott's fracture *Inclusion in this rubric requires* both *of the following:* (a) Trauma to the bone (b) *One* of the following: (i) X-ray evidence of a fracture (ii) Visible or palpable deformity or crepitus involving the bone *Consider:* (*327*, **929-**) Bruise, contusion	823, 824
311	829-	**All other specified, or ill-defined fractures** *Inclusion in this rubric requires* both *of the following:* (a) Trauma to the bone (b) *One* of the following: (i) X-ray evidence of a fracture (ii) Visible or palpable deformity or crepitus involving the bone *Consider:* (*327*, **929-**) Bruise, contusion; (*333*, **959-**) Other injury or trauma	807.2–807.6, 808, 809, 811, 817–819, 822, 827–829

Dislocations

312	836-	**Acute damage to meniscus of knee** *excl.* chronic damage to meniscus (*244*, **717-**) *Inclusion in this rubric requires:* An initial injury to the meniscus which occurred no longer than one month previously and *one* of the following: (a) Demonstration of meniscus tear at surgery, arthroscopy, or X-ray (b) *All* of the following: (i) Locking or giving way of the knee (ii) Pain in knee (iii) Swelling of knee (iv) Tenderness over joint space *Consider:* (*244*, **717-**) Chronic damage to meniscus; (*316*, **844-**) Sprain of knee	836.0–836.2

Position no.	ICHPPC code	List of diseases, disorders, and health problems, with inclusion criteria	Comparable ICD-9 codes

313   **839-**   **All other dislocations and subluxations**   830–835, 836.3–836.6, 837–839

Inclusion in this rubric requires both *of the following:*
(a) A history of trauma to the joint
(b) *One* of the following:
   (i) X-ray evidence of dislocation or subluxation
   (ii) Palpable or visible dislocation deformity
Consider: (*314*, **840-** to *321*, **848-**) Sprains and strains

Sprains and strains (of joints, muscles and ligaments)

314   **840-**   **Shoulder, upper arm, elbow, forearm**   840, 841
Inclusion in this rubric requires both *of the following*
(a) Stretch injury of the affected part
(b) Pain aggravated by stretching or tensing the affected structure

315   **842-**   **Wrist, hand, finger**   842
Inclusion in this rubric requires both *of the following:*
(a) Stretch injury of the affected part
(b) Pain aggravated by stretching or tensing the affected structure

316   **844-**   **Knee (lower leg)**   844
Inclusion in this rubric requires both *of the following:*
(a) Stretch injury of the affected part
(b) Pain aggravated by stretching or tensing the affected structure

317   **8450**   **Ankle**   845.0
Inclusion in this rubric requires both *of the following:*
(a) Stretch injury of the affected part
(b) Pain aggravated by stretching or tensing the affected structure

318   **8451**   **Foot, toe**   845.1
Inclusion in this rubric requires both *of the following:*
(a) Stretch injury of the affected part
(b) Pain aggravated by stretching or tensing the affected structure

Position no.	ICHPPC code	List of diseases, disorders, and health problems, with inclusion criteria	Comparable ICD-9 codes
319	8470	**Neck** incl. whiplash Inclusion in this rubric requires both of the following: (a) Stretch injury of the affected part (b) Pain aggravated by stretching or tensing the affected structure	847.0
320	8478	**Rest of vertebral column** incl. sacroiliac region, coccyx Inclusion in this rubric requires both of the following: (a) Stretch injury of the affected part (b) Pain aggravated by stretching or tensing the affected structure	846, 847.1–847.9
321	848-	**All other sprains and strains** incl. ill-defined Inclusion in this rubric requires both of the following: (a) Stretch injury of the affected part (b) Pain aggravated by stretching or tensing the affected structure	843, 848

Other trauma

322	850-	**Head injury, concussion, intracranial injury, without skull fracture** excl. psychological effects (86, 316-); late effects (322, 908-) Inclusion in this rubric requires both of the following: (a) Trauma to the head (b) Abnormal neurological symptoms or signs Consider: (301, 802-) Fractured skull; (327, 929-) Bruise, contusion; (333, 959-) Other injury or trauma	850–854
323	889-	**Laceration, open wound, traumatic amputation** incl. animal bite; injuries to teeth and eardrum; puncture wound As defined in the diagnostic title Consider: (333, 959-) if wound infected	870–897
324	—	(Deleted)	
325	910-	**Insect bite and sting** As defined in the diagnostic title	pt. 910–919, 989.5

Position no.	ICHPPC code	List of diseases, disorders, and health problems, with inclusion criteria	Comparable ICD-9 codes
326	**918-**	**Abrasion, scratch, blister** *incl.* eye abrasion *As defined in the diagnostic title* *Consider:* (*333*, **959-**) if wound infected	pt. 910–919
327	**929-**	**Bruise, contusion, crushing with intact skin surface** *incl.* contusion of eye; hematoma *excl.* internal organ injury (*333*, **959-**); spontaneous subconjunctival hemorrhage (*99*, **378-**) *As defined in the diagnostic title*	920–929
328	**949-**	**Burns, scalds—all degrees** *incl.* burns of eye; chemical; electrical; radiation *As defined in the diagnostic title*	940–949
329	**912-**	**Foreign body in superficial tissues** *excl.* foreign body in eye (*330*, **930-**); residual or old foreign body in tissues, foreign body granuloma (*234*, **728-**) *As defined in the diagnostic title*	pt. 910–919
330	**930-**	**Foreign body in eye** *incl.* adnexa *excl.* residual or old foreign body in the eye (*99*, **378-**) *As defined in the diagnostic title*	930
331	**939-**	**Foreign body entering through orifice** *excl.* eye (*330*, **930-**) *As defined in the diagnostic title*	931–939
332	**908-**	**Late effects of trauma** *incl.* deformaties; disabilities; scarring *excl.* psychological (*86*, **316-**); non-union, malunion of fracture (*246*, **739-**) *As defined in the diagnostic title*	905–909
333	**959-**	**Other injury or trauma** *incl.* early complication of trauma; infected wound; internal injury of chest, abdomen, and pelvis; laceration and other injury to nerve; multiple trauma *As defined in the diagnostic title* *Note*: For suicide or attempted suicide, code the nature of the self-inflicted injury or adverse effect in addition to any known underlying emotion or social problem	860–869, 900–904, 950–959

Position no.	ICHPPC code	List of diseases, disorders, and health problems, with inclusion criteria	Comparable ICD-9 codes

Adverse effects

334	**977-**	**Poisoning by medicinal agent, accidental or deliberate overdose** *As defined in the diagnostic title*	960–979
(377)	**9952**	**Adverse effect of medical agent correctly administered in proper dosage** May also code the nature of the adverse effect *excl.* addiction or habituation (*83*, **3048**); dermatitis (*214*, **692-**); reaction to immunization and transfusion (*336*, **998-**); allergy and anaphylaxis (*378*, **9950**), anesthetic shock (*378*, **9950**) *Inclusion in this rubric requires:* Symptoms or signs thought to be caused by the use of medication, rather than due to disease or injury	995.2
335	**989-**	**Toxic effects of other substances** *incl.* carbon monoxide; industrial materials; lead; poisonous plants *excl.* burns—internal or external (*328*, **949-**); contact dermatitis (*214*, **692-**); respiratory toxic effects (*147*, **519-**) *Inclusion in this rubric requires:* Symptoms or signs thought to be caused by exposure to toxic non-medicinal substances	980–989 ex. pt. 989.5
336	**998-**	**Complications of surgery and medical treatment** *incl.* complications of prostheses, devices, and implants; immunization and transfusion reactions; post-operative wound infection, hemorrhage, and disruption *excl.* adverse effects of drugs (*377*, **9952**); adverse effects of diagnostic and therapeutic X-rays (*337*, **994-**); infected traumatic wound (*333*, **959-**) *As defined in the diagnostic title*	996–999
337	**994-**	**Adverse effects of physical factors** *incl.* cold (incl. chilblains; drowning; heat; lightning; motion; pressure; radiation (natural or industrial, diagnostic, or therapeutic) *excl.* burns due to radiation (*328*, **949-**); snowblindness (*99*, **378-**); sunburn (*214*, **692-**) *As defined in the diagnostic title*	990–994
(378)	**9950**	**Certain adverse effects not elsewhere classified** *incl.* allergic edema; allergic reaction NOS; anaphylactic shock; anesthetic shock; angioneurotic edema *Inclusion criteria for this rubric are not listed*	995 ex. 995.2

Position no.	ICHPPC code	List of diseases, disorders, and health problems, with inclusion criteria	Comparable ICD-9 codes

XVIII. SUPPLEMENTARY CLASSIFICATION

Preventive medicine

338	V70-	**Medical examination** (where this is considered to be a reason for the contact) *incl.* care of well child or infant; complete or partial checkups; cytology smear; examination or investigation to exclude specific disease; health screening; malingering; normal variation; preoperative examination; 'worried well' *Inclusion in this rubric requires:* A medical examination for the purpose of health screening or health maintenance with *one* of the following: (a) No symptoms presented and no problems found (b) No symptoms presented, but problem(s) found (double code the problem(s)) *Consider:* (*339*, **V01-**) if contact with disease; (*341*, **V14-** and *342*, **V10-**) if screening because of high-risk situation; (*354*, **V654**) Advice, health instruction and education if no medical examination is involved	V20, V21, V28, V30–V39, V65.2, V65.5, V70, V71, V72 ex. V72.7, V73–V82
339	V01-	**Contacts and carriers (suspected or proven) of infective or parasitic disease** *incl.* prophylactic therapy *excl.* rheumatic fever prophylaxis (*108*, **390-**) *Inclusion in this rubric requires* one *of the following:* (a) Contact with a person or fomite harboring pathogenic organisms (b) Carrier (suspected or proven) of pathogenic organisms, without signs or symptoms of the illness caused by those organisms (c) Need for prophylactic therapy other than immunizations	V01, V02, V07, ex. V07.1
340	V03-	**Prophylactic immunization, inoculation and vaccination** *As defined in the diagnostic title*	V03–V06
341	V14-	**Observation and care of patient on high-risk medication** Requires: additional code for primary diagnosis *As defined in the diagnostic title*	No equivalent ICD-9 code

Position no.	ICHPPC code	List of diseases, disorders, and health problems, with inclusion criteria	Comparable ICD-9 codes
342	**V10-**	**Observation and care of other high-risk patients** *incl.* family history of certain diseases; occupational hazards; patient-care management of prosthetic devices and implants; personal history of certain diseases; status post-surgery *Inclusion in this rubric requires:* Specification by the health care provider that there is a high risk for a condition for which the patient is being observed Requires: Additional code for primary diagnosis	V10–V13, V15–V19, V42–V46 (ex. V45.5)

Family planning

343	**V252**	**Sterilization of male or female** *Inclusion in this rubric requires:* Provision of, or arrangements for, a procedure undertaken with the explicit intention of terminating fertility *Consider:* (*347*, **V256**) Discussion of sterilization *Note:* Pap smear should be double coded (*338*, **V70-**)	pt. V25.0, pt. V25.4
344	**V255**	**Oral contraceptive** *Inclusion in this rubric requires:* Discussion, prescription, or examination in connection with an oral contraceptive *Consider:* (*347*, **V256**) General contraceptive advice *Note:* Code the contraceptive method to be commenced or continued, not that being discontinued, unless no further contraception is to be used Pap smear should be coded separately (*338*, **V70-**)	pt. V25.0, pt. V25.4
345	**V251**	**Intrauterine device** *Inclusion in this rubric requires:* Consultation regarding insertion of, or follow-up examination, investigation, or removal of an intrauterine device *Consider:* (*347*, **V256**) General contraceptive advice *Note:* Code the contraceptive method to be commenced or continued, not that being discontinued, unless no further contraception is to be used Pap smear should be coded separately (*338*, **V70-**)	V25.1, pt. V25.4, V45.5

Position no.	ICHPPC code	List of diseases, disorders, and health problems, with inclusion criteria	Comparable ICD-9 codes
346	**V253**	**Other method of contraception** *Inclusion in this rubric requires:* Discussion, advice, examination in regard to provision of other methods of contraception, including condom, pessary, foams, but excluding oral contraceptives and intrauterine device *Consider:* (*347*, **V256**) General contraceptive advice *Note:* Code the contraceptive method to be commenced or continued, not that being discontinued, unless no further contraception is to be used Pap smear should be coded separately (*338*, **V70-**)	V25.3, pt. V25.4, V25.8, V25.9
347	**V256**	**General contraceptive advice** *incl.* advice about sterilization or therapeutic abortion *Inclusion in this rubric requires* A general discussion with the patient about contraception, therapeutic abortion, or sterilization, with or without any associated examination, counseling, or health education, but without provision of any specific method *Note:* The actual provision of any method, including follow-up care, is classified as (*343*, **V252**), (*344*, **V255**), (*345*, **V251**), (*346*, **V253**) Pap smear should be coded separately (*338*, **V70-**)	pt. V25.0

Administrative procedures

348	**V680**	**Letters, forms, certificates, and prescriptions** with need for additional examination or interview of patient *excl.* prescription for oral contraceptive (*344*, **V255**); letters and reports relating to a third party (*355*, **V651**) *Inclusion in this rubric requires:* The preparation of a written document where the underlying problem is not coded elsewhere	V68 (ex. pt. V68.8)
349	**V683**	**Referral of patient** without need for examination or interview *Inclusion in this rubric requires:* Referral to another health care provider, where the underlying problem is not coded elsewhere	pt. V68.8

Position no.	ICHPPC code	List of diseases, disorders, and health problems, with inclusion criteria	Comparable ICD-9 codes

Maternal and child health care

350	**V223**	**The diagnosis of pregnancy** *Inclusion in this rubric requires:* Confirmation of the existence of a pregnancy by history, examination, or other investigation	pt. V22.0–V22.2
351	**V220**	**Prenatal care or incidentally noted to be pregnant** Requires: Additional code for: associated non-obstetrical condition (*passim*), complication of pregnancy (*199*, **642-**), (*202*, **648-**) (*197-*, **640-**), (*198*, **6466**) *As defined in the diagnostic title*	pt. V22.0–V22.2, V23
352	**V24-**	**Postpartum care** (of mother) *excl.* suppression of lactation (*205*, **676-**) *As defined in the diagnostic title*	V24

Miscellaneous

353	**V50-**	**Medical or surgical procedure without reported diagnosis** *incl.* circumcision without disease; piercing of ears; surgical assist *Inclusion in this rubric requires:* The doctor–problem contact is restricted to a medical or surgical procedure where no diagnosis is recorded and which is not coded elsewhere *Consider:* (*354*, **V654**) Advice, health instruction, and education when a procedure is discussed, but not performed	V50, V51
354	**V654**	**Advice, health instruction and education** *incl.* class instruction *excl.* contraceptive instruction (*347*, **V256**) *Inclusion in this rubric requires:* Advice or instruction not related to a specific condition classifiable elsewhere *Consider:* (*338*, **V70-**) if medical examination is performed	V26.3, V26.4, V65.3, V65.4

Position no.	ICHPPC code	List of diseases, disorders, and health problems, with inclusion criteria	Comparable ICD-9 codes
355	**V651**	**Problems external to patient** *incl.* blood donor; consulting for another (e.g. sick relative); manifestation of anxiety in a third party *Inclusion in this rubric requires* one *of the following:* (a) A problem which does not affect the person taking part in the encounter, but rather someone else: the 'presenting patient', is acting as messenger (b) Donation of blood for the benefit of another or as a credit for future use by the donor *Consider: (358,* **V614-**) if the outside illness is a problem for the 'presenting patient'	V59, V65.1

Social, marital, and family problems and maladjustments

Note: This section is for social problems and maladjustments (inside or outside the family) which have been discussed with the patient and which are accepted by him as a significant problem. More than one code may be applied to a patient. These codes may be used alone to describe the substance or content of an encounter, or may be used as additional codes to show the interdependence between organic or mental problems and the social milieu of the patient. The classification of social problems and maladjustments in primary health care involves a bi-axial model. One axis describes the psychological reaction forms and is classified in Chapter V. The second axis describes the actual content of the social problem and is classified in this chapter. Psychosocial problems should be classified on both axes whenever possible. This section excludes contact with person acting as emissary for another person who is experiencing problems (*355*, **V651**)

356	**V602**	**Economic problem, poverty** *Inclusion in this rubric requires:* A problem concerning the economic circumstances of the patient or his family	V60.2
357	**V600**	**Housing problem** *Inclusion in this rubric requires:* A problem concerning the housing conditions of a patient or his family	V60.0, V60.1

Position no.	ICHPPC code	List of diseases, disorders, and health problems, with inclusion criteria	Comparable ICD-9 codes
358	**V614**	**Problem of caring for sick person** (e.g. alcoholic family member) *excl.* patient lacking person able to render care (*366*, **V642**) *Inclusion in this rubric requires:* A problem concerning the patient's care of a sick person *Note:* This includes problems of care or treatment in addition to the emotional or physical strain on the patient in coping with a sick person. It excludes the receipt of advice or prescription on behalf of the sick person (*355*, **V651**)	V61.4
359	**V611**	**Marital problem** *incl.* problems of the relationship between a man and a woman, whether married or not *excl.* problems limited to sexual activity (*79*, **3027**) *Inclusion in this rubric requires:* A problem involving the relationship between the patient and a sexual partner (incl. homosexual) whether legally married or not *Consider:* (*79*, **3027**) Psychogenic disorder of sexual function if the problem is primarily sexual	V61.1
360	**V612**	**Parent–child problem** *incl.* concern about behavior of child; problems related to adopted or foster child; child abuse, battered child, child neglect *Inclusion in this rubric requires:* A problem involving the relationship between parent(s) and child(ren) *Note:* The patient may be a child to age 18 or a parent with a child to age 18. If the child is aged 18 or more, code (*361*, **V613**). If the patient's child is age 18 or more, code (*363*, **V619**)	V61.2
361	**V613**	**Problems with aged parents or in-laws** *Inclusion in this rubric requires:* A problem experienced by an adult (age 18 or over) with his parents or in-laws *Note:* For parents with problems with children over age 18, code (*363*, **V619**)	V61.3

Position no.	ICHPPC code	List of diseases, disorders, and health problems, with inclusion criteria	Comparable ICD-9 codes
362	**V610**	**Family disruption,** with or without divorce, affecting the couple or others *excl.* bereavement (*77,* **308-**) *Inclusion in this rubric requires:* A problem regarding the physical disruption of the family, e.g. the separation of one, some, or all of its members through divorce, disappearance, death, or any other long-standing physical absence (job, military service, etc.) *Consider:* (*359,* **V611**) Marital problem; (*360,* **V612**) Parent-child problem; (*361,* **V613**) Aged parent problem; (*363,* **V619**) Other family problem	V61.0
363	**V619**	**Other problem of the family relationship NEC** *Inclusion criteria for this rubric are not listed*	V61.5, V61.7–V61.9
364	**V623**	**Educational problem** *excl.* specific learning disturbances (*74,* **315-**) *Inclusion in this rubric requires* one *of the following:* (a) A problem with formal education in school or in other educational institutions (b) A problem which is related to one or more of the following: the intellectual, cognitive, or social aspects of the educational environment (c) A problem which derives from insufficient or inappropriate education	V62.3
365	**V616**	**Pregnancy out of wedlock (illegitimate pregnancy), illegitimacy** *Inclusion in this rubric requires:* A problem arising from a pregnancy conceived outside of the legal relationship of a marriage *Consider:* (*365,* **V619**) if unwanted pregnancy within or without marriage	V61.6
366	**V624**	**Social maladjustment** *incl.* social isolation, persecution, cultural deprivation, political, religious, or sex discrimination *Inclusion in this rubric requires:* Difficulties coping with the social environment NOS *Note:* This maladjustment may result from a social system which does not permit adaptation by the patient	V60.3–V60.6, V62.4

Position no.	ICHPPC code	List of diseases, disorders, and health problems, with inclusion criteria	Comparable ICD-9 codes
367	**V620**	**Occupational problem** *incl.* career choice problem or frustration; difficulties at work or in adjusting to work situation; unemployment *Inclusion in this rubric requires:* A problem which concerns the occupational situation	V62.0–V62.2
368	**V627**	**Phase of life social problem NEC** *Inclusion in this rubric requires:* A problem concerning adjustment to a certain phase of life (e.g. childhood, adolescence, marriage, change of life, retirement, old age) *Consider:* (*77*, **308-**) Transient situational disturbance, bereavement	pt. V62.8
(370)	**V625**	**Legal problem** *incl.* imprisonment; legal investigations; litigation; prosecution *Inclusion in this rubric requires:* A problem concerning a conflict between the patient and the legal system	V62.5
369	**V629**	**Other social problems** *incl.* refusal of treatment for reasons of religion or conscience *Inclusion criteria for this rubric are not listed*	V60.8, V60.9, V62.2–V62.9 (ex. pt. V62.8)
370	**V625-**	(See after position number 368)	
371	**V999**	**All other problems not classifiable in codes 008- to V629** *incl.* disfigurement or cosmetic problem NOS; other supplementary classification; options detailed in ICD *Inclusion criteria for this rubric are not listed*	V07.1, V14, V25.4, V26 (ex. V26.3, V26.4) V27, V40, V41, V47–V49, V52–V58, V63–V64, V65.0, V65.8, V65.9, V66, V67, V72.7
372	**0994**	(See after position number 23)	
373	**5997**	(See after position number 173)	
374	**6254**	(See after position number 188)	
375	**7900**	(See after position number 298)	
376	**7950**	(See after position number 298, 375, 51)	
377	**9952**	(See after position number 334)	
378	**9950**	(See after position number 337)	

Appendix 1: Condensed titles for machine processing and computer printouts

This list of condensed diagnostic titles is designed for machine processing and computer printouts. Each title contains a maximum of 35 letters and spaces. It is necessary to refer to the tabular section for the full content of each rubric. The following abbreviations and symbols are used:

&	and, and/or
( )	out of sequence
EXCL	excluding
INCL	including
NEC	not elsewhere classified
NOS	not otherwise specified
NYD	not yet diagnosed
WO	without
W/WO	with or without

Position no.	ICHPPC code	Condensed title

I. INFECTIVE & PARASITIC DISEASES

1	008-	PROVEN INFECTIOUS INTESTINE DISEASE
2	009-	PRESUMED INFECTIOUS INTESTIN DISEAS
3	—	(Deleted)
4	011-	TUBERCULOSIS
5	5119	(See after position number 141)
6	033-	WHOOPING COUGH
7	034-	STREP THROAT, SCARLET FEV, ERYSIPELAS
8	045-	POLIO & CNS ENTEROVIRAL DISEASES
9	052-	CHICKENPOX
10	053-	HERPES ZOSTER
11	054-	HERPES SIMPLEX
12	055-	MEASLES
13	056-	RUBELLA
14	057-	OTHER VIRAL EXANTHEMS
15	070-	INFECTIOUS HEPATITIS
16	072-	MUMPS
17	075-	INFECTIOUS MONONUCLEOSIS
18	077-	VIRAL CONJUNCTIVITIS
19	0781	WARTS, ALL SITES
20	0799	VIRAL INFECTION NOS
21	084-	MALARIA
22	090-	SYPHILIS, ALL SITES & STAGES
23	098-	GONORREA, ALL SITES
(372)	0994	NON-SPECIFIC URETHRITIS
24	110-	DERMATOPHYTOSIS & DERMATOMYCOSIS
25	112-	MONILIASIS EXCL UROGENITAL
26	1121	MONILIASIS, UROGENITAL, PROVEN
27	1310	TRICHOMONIASIS, UROGENITAL, PROVEN
28	127-	OXYURIASIS, PINWORMS, HELMINTH NEC
29	132-	PEDICULOSIS & OTHER INFESTATIONS
30	133-	SCABIES & OTHER ACARIASIS
31	136-	OTHER INFECT/PARASITIC DISEASES NEC

Position no.	ICHPPC code	Condensed title

II. NEOPLASMS

Malignant neoplasms

32	151-	MALIG NEOPL GASTROINTESTINAL TRACT
33	162-	MALIGNANT NEOPL RESPIRATORY TRACT
34	173-	MALIG NEOPL SKIN/SUBCUTANEOUS TISSU
35	174-	MALIGNANT NEOPLASM BREAST
36	180-	MALIG NEOPL FEMALE GENITAL TRACT
37	188-	MALIG NEOPL URINARY & MALE GENITAL
38	201-	HODGKINS DISEASE, LYMPHOMA, LEUKEMIA
39	199-	OTHER MALIGNANT NEOPLASMS NEC

Benign neoplasms

40	214-	LIPOMA, ANY SITE
41	216-	BENIGN NEOPLASM SKIN
42	217-	BENIGN NEOPLASM BREAST
43	218-	BENIGN NEOPLASM UTERUS
44	228-	HEMANGIOMA & LYMPHANGIOMA
45	229-	OTHER BENIGN NEOPLASMS NEC

Unspecified neoplasms

46	239-	NEOPL NYD AS BENIGN OR MALIGNANT

Position no.	ICHPPC code	Condensed title

III. ENDOCR, NUTRIT, METABOL DISEAS

47	240-	NONTOXIC GOITER & NODULE
48	242-	THYROTOXICOSIS W/WO GOITER
49	244-	HYPOTHYROIDISM, MYXEDEMA, CRETINISM
50	250-	DIABETES MELLITUS
51	7902	(See after position number 294)
52	260-	AVITAMIN & NUTRITIONAL DISORDER NEC
53	7833	(See after position number 294)
54	274-	GOUT
55	278-	OBESITY
56	272-	LIPID METABOLISM DISORDERS
57	279-	OTHER ENDOCR, NUTRITN, METABOL DISORD

Position no.	ICHPPC code	Condensed title

IV. BLOOD DISEASES

58	280-	IRON DEFICIENCY ANEMIA
59	281-	PERNICIOUS & OTHER DEFICIENC ANEMIA
60	282-	HEREDITARY HEMOLYTIC ANEMIAS
61	285-	ANEMIA, OTHER/UNSPECIFIED
62	287-	PURPURA, HEMORRHAG & COAGULAT DEFECT
63	2891	LYMPHADENITIS, CHRONIC/NONSPECIFIC
64	288-	ABNORMAL WHITE CELLS
65	2899	BLOOD/BLOOD FORMING ORGAN DISOR NEC

Position no.	ICHPPC code	Condensed title

V. MENTAL DISORDERS

Psychoses except alcoholic

66	294-	ORGANIC PSYCHOSIS EXCL ALCOHOLIC
67	295-	SCHIZOPHRENIA, ALL TYPES
68	296-	AFFECTIVE PSYCHOSES
69	298-	PSYCHOSIS, OTHER/NOS EXCL ALCOHOLIC

Neuroses

70	3000	ANXIETY DISORDER
71	3001	HYSTERICAL & HYPOCHONDRIAC DISORDER
72	3004	DEPRESSIVE DISORDER
73	3009	NEUROSIS, OTHER/UNSPECIFIED

Other mental, psycholog disorders

74	315-	SPECIFIC LEARNING DISTURBANCE
75	3074	INSOMNIA & OTHER SLEEP DISORDERS
76	3078	TENSION HEADACHE
77	308-	TRANSIEN SITUAT DISTURB, ADJ REACT
78	312-	BEHAVIOR DISORDERS NEC
79	3027	SEXUAL PROBLEMS
80	3031	ALCOHOL ABUSE & ALCOHOLIC PSYCHOSIS
81	3050	ACUTE ALCOHOLIC INTOXICATION
82	3051	TOBACCO ABUSE
83	3048	OTHER DRUG ABUSE, HABIT, ADDICTION
84	301-	PERSONALITY & CHARACTER DISORDERS
85	317-	MENTAL RETARDATION
86	316-	OTHER MENTAL & PSYCHOLOGIC DISORDER

Position no.	ICHPPC code	Condensed title

VII. CIRCULATORY SYSTEM DISEASES

Heart diseases

108	390-	RHEUMATIC FEVER/HEART DISEASE
109	410-	AC MYOCARD INFARCT/SUBAC ISCHEMIA
110	412-	CHRONIC ISCHEMIC HEART DISEASE
111	424-	(See after position number 117)
112	428-	HEART FAILURE, RIGHT/LEFT SIDED
113	4273	ATRIAL FIBRILLATION OR FLUTTER
114	4270	PAROXYSMAL TACHYCARDIA
115	4276	ECTOPIC BEATS, ALL TYPES
116		(See after position number 264)
117	416-	PULMONARY HEART DISEASE
(111)	424-	DISEAS HEART VALV NON-RHEUM, NOS, NYD
118	429-	OTHER HEART DISEASES NEC

Blood pressure problems

119	7962	(See after position numbers 298 and (375), (51), (376))
120	401-	HYPERTENSION, UNCOMPLICATED
121	402-	HYPERTENSION INVOLVING TARGET ORGAN
122	—	(Deleted)

Vascular system diseases

123	435-	TRANSIENT CEREBRAL ISCHEMIA
124	438-	OTHER CEREBROVASCULAR DISEASE
125	440-	ATHEROSCLEROSIS EXCL HEART & BRAIN
126	443-	OTHER ARTERIAL DISEAS EXCL ANEURYSM
127	415-	PULMONARY EMBOLISM & INFARCTION
128	451-	PHLEBITIS & THROMBOPHLEBITIS
129	454-	VARICOSE VEINS OF LEGS
130	455-	HEMORRHOIDS
131	4580	POSTURAL HYPOTENSION
132	459-	OTHER PERIPHERAL VESSEL DISEASES

VIII. RESPIRATORY SYSTEM DISEASES

IX. DIGESTIVE SYSTEM DISEASES

Position no.	ICHPPC code	Condensed title

X. GENITOURINARY SYSTEM DISEASES

Urinary system diseases

168	580-	GLOMERULONEPHRITIS, ACUTE & CHRONIC
169	5901	PYELONEPHRITIS & PYELITIS, ACUTE
170	595-	CYSTITIS & URINARY INFECTION NOS
171	592-	URINARY SYSTEM CALCULUS, ALL TYPES
172	597-	URETHRITIS NOS, NEC
173	5936	ORTHOSTATIC ALBUMINURIA
(373)	5997	HEMATURIA NOS
174	598-	OTHER URINARY SYSTEM DISEASES NEC

Male genital organ diseases

175	600-	BENIGN PROSTATIC HYPERTROPHY
176	601-	PROSTATIS & SEMINAL VESICULITIS
177	603-	HYDROCELE
178	604-	ORCHITIS & EPIDIDYMITIS
179	605-	REDUND PREPUCE, PHIMOSIS & BALANITIS
180	607-	OTHER MALE GENITAL ORGAN DISEASES

Breast diseases

181	610-	CHRONIC CYSTIC BREAST DISEASE
182	611-	OTHER BREAST DISEASES

Female genital organ diseases

183	614-	PELVIC INFLAMMATORY DISEASE
184	622-	CERVICITIS & CERVICAL EROSION
185	6161	VAGINITIS NOS, VULVITIS
186	618-	UTEROVAGINAL PROLAPSE
187	627-	MENOPAUSAL SYMPTOMS & POST MENO BLEED
188	6254	PREMENSTRUAL TENSION SYNDROME
(374)	6250	NON-PSYCH VAGINISMUS & DYSPAREUNIA

Position no.	ICHPPC code	Condensed title

Disorders of menstruation

189	6260	ABSENT, SCANTY, RARE MENSTRUATION
190	6262	EXCESSIVE MENSTRUATION
191	6253	PAINFUL MENSTRUATION
192	—	(Deleted)
193	6269	INTERMENSTR BLEEDING
194	629-	OTHER FEMALE GENITAL ORGAN DISEASES

Fertility problems

| *195* | 606- | STERILITY & REDUCED FERTILITY |

Position no.	ICHPPC code	Condensed title

XII. SKIN, SUBCUTANEOUS TISSU DISEAS

207	680-	BOIL & CELLULITIS INCL FINGR & TOE
208	—	(Deleted)
209	683-	LYMPHADENITIS, ACUTE
210	684-	IMPETIGO
211	685-	OTHER INFECTIONS SKIN/SUBCUTANEOUS
212	690-	SEBORRHEIC DERMATITIS
213	6918	ECZEMA & ALLERGIC DERMATITIS
214	692-	CONTACT & OTHER DERMATITIS NEC
215	6910	DIAPER RASH
216	6963	PITYRIASIS ROSEA
217	6961	PSORIASIS W/WO ARTHROPATHY
218	698-	PRURITIS & RELATED CONDITIONS
219	700-	CORNS & CALLOSITIES
220	7062	SEBACEOUS CYST
221	703-	INGROWN TOENAIL & NAIL DISEASE NEC
222	704-	ALOPECIA & OTHER HAIR DISEASES
223	705-	POMPHOLYX & SWEAT GLAND DIS NEC
224	7061	ACNE
225	707-	CHRONIC SKIN ULCER
226	708-	URTICARIA
227	709-	OTHER SKIN & SUBCUTANE TISSU DISEAS

Position no.	ICHPPC code	Condensed title

XV. PERINATAL MORBIDITY & MORTALITY

253   778-   ALL PERINATAL CONDITIONS

XVI. SIGN, SYMPTOM, ILL DEFINED COND

Central & peripheral nerv system

Cardiovascular & lymphatic system

Respiratory system

Gastrointestinal system & abdomen

Position no.	ICHPPC code	Condensed title

Genitourinary system

280	7881	DYSURIA
281	7883	ENURESIS, INCONTINENCE
282	—	(*Deleted*)
283	7884	FREQUENCY OF URINATION
284	—	(*Deleted*)
285	—	(*Deleted*)
286	7295	(See after position number 234)
287	—	(*Deleted*)
288	7194	(See after position number 230)
289	7190	(See after position numbers 230, 288)

General signs & symptoms

290	7808	EXCESSIVE SWEATING
291	7806	FEVER OF UNDETERMINED CAUSE
292	7821	RASH & OTHER NONSPECIFIC SKIN ERUPT
293	7832	WEIGHT LOSS
294	7834	LACK OF EXPECTED PHYSIOLOG DEVELOP
(53)	7833	FEEDING PROBLEM BABY OR ELDERLY
295	7807	MALAISE, FATIGUE, TIREDNESS
296	7822	MASS & LOCALIZED SWELLING NOS/NYD
297	797-	SENILITY WITHOUT PSYCHOSIS

Position no.	ICHPPC code	Condensed title

Unexplained abnormal results

Urinanalysis

298	791-	ABNORMAL URINE TEST NEC

Hematology

(375)	7900	HEMATOLOGICAL ABNORMALITY NEC

Blood chemistry

(51)	7902	ABNORMAL UNEXPLAINED BIOCHEM TEST

Other abnormal results

(376)	7950	NON-SPECIFIC ABNORMAL PAP SMEAR
(119)	7962	ELEVATED BLOOD PRESSURE
299	793-	OTHER UNEXPLAINED ABNORMAL RESULTS

Sign, symptom, ill defined cond NEC

300	7889	SIGN, SYMPTOM, ILL DEFINED COND NEC

Position no.	ICHPPC code	Condensed title

XVII. INJURIES & ADVERSE EFFECTS

Fractures

301	802-	FRACTURE SKULL & FACIAL BONES
302	805-	FRACTURE VERTEBRAL COLUMN
303	807-	FRACTURE RIBS
304	810-	FRACTURE CLAVICLE
305	812-	FRACTURE HUMERUS
306	813-	FRACTURE RADIUS/ULNA
307	814-	FRACT (META)CARPAL & (META)TARSAL
308	816-	FRACTURE PHALANGES FOOT/HAND
309	820-	FRACTURE FEMUR
310	823-	FRACTURE TIBIA/FIBULA
311	829-	FRACTURE ALL OTHER SITES NEC

Dislocations & subluxations

312	836-	ACUTE DAMAGE KNEE MENISCUS
313	839-	DISLOC/SUBLUX OTHER SITES NEC

Sprains & strains

314	840-	SPRAIN/STRAIN SHOULDER & ARM
315	842-	SPRAIN/STRAIN WRIST, HAND, FINGERS
316	844-	SPRAIN/STRAIN KNEE & LOWER LEG
317	8450	SPRAIN/STRAIN ANKLE
318	8451	SPRAIN/STRAIN FOOT & TOES
319	8470	SPRAIN/STRAIN NECK
320	8478	SPRAIN/STRAIN VERTEBRAL EXCL NECK
321	848-	SPRAIN & STRAIN ALL OTHER SITES NEC

Position no.	ICHPPC code	Condensed title

Other traumas

322	850-	CONCUSSION & INTRACRANIAL INJURY
323	889-	LACERAT/OPEN WOUND/TRAUM AMPUTATN
324	—	(Deleted)
325	910-	INSECT BITES & STINGS
326	918-	ABRASION, SCRATCH, BLISTER
327	929-	BRUISE, CONTUSION, CRUSHING
328	949-	BURNS & SCALDS, ALL DEGREES
329	912-	FOREIGN BODY IN TISSUES
330	930-	FOREIGN BODY IN EYE
331	939-	FOREIGN BODY ENTERING THRU ORIFICE
332	908-	LATE EFFECT OF TRAUMA
333	959-	OTHER INJURIES & TRAUMA

Adverse effects

334	977-	OVERDOS MEDICIN ACCID OR DELIBERAT
(377)	9952	ADVERS EFFECT MEDICIN PROPER DOSE
335	989-	ADVERSE EFFECTS OF OTHER CHEMICALS
336	998-	SURGERY & MEDICAL CARE COMPLICATION
337	994-	ADVERSE EFFECTS OF PHYSICAL FACTORS
(378)	9950	OTHER ADVERSE EFFECTS NEC

Position no.	ICHPPC code	Condensed title

SUPPLEMENTARY CLASSIFICATION

Preventive medicine

338	V70-	MEDICAL EXAM
339	V01-	CONTAC/CARRIER, INFEC/PARASIT DIS
340	V03-	PROPHYLACTIC IMMUNIZATION
341	V14-	OBSERV/CARE PT ON HI RISK MEDICAT
342	V10-	OBSERV/CARE OTHER HI RISK PATIENT

Family planning

343	V252	STERILIZATION OF MALE OR FEMALE
344	V255	ORAL CONTRACEPTIVES
345	V251	INTRAUTERINE DEVICES
346	V253	OTHER CONTRACEPTIVE METHODS
347	V256	GENERAL CONTRACEPTIVE GUIDANCE

Administrative procedures

348	V680	LETTER, FORMS, PRESCRIPTION WO EXAM
349	V683	REFERRAL WO EXAM OR INTERVIEW

Maternal & child health care

350	V223	DIAGNOSING PREGNANCY
351	V220	PRENATAL CARE
352	V24-	POSTNATAL CARE

Miscellaneous

353	V50-	MED/SURG PROCEDURE WO DIAGNOSIS
354	V654	ADVICE & HEALTH INSTRUCTION
355	V651	PROBLEMS EXTERNAL TO PATIENT

Position no.	ICHPPC code	Condensed title

Social, marital, family problems

356	V602	ECONOMIC PROBLEM
357	V600	HOUSING PROBLEM
358	V614	MEDICAL CARE PROBLEM
359	V611	MARITAL PROBLEM
360	V612	PARENT & CHILD PROBLEM
361	V613	AGED PARENT OR INLAW PROBLEM
362	V610	FAMILY DISRUPTION W/WO DIVORCE
363	V619	OTHER FAMILY PROBLEMS
364	V623	EDUCATIONAL PROBLEM
365	V616	PREGNANCY OUT OF WEDLOCK
366	V624	SOCIAL MALADJUSTMENT
367	V620	OCCUPATIONAL PROBLEM
368	V627	PHASE-OF-LIFE PROBLEM NEC
(370)	V625	LEGAL PROBLEM
369	V629	OTHER SOCIAL PROBLEM
370	V625	(See after position number 368)

Other problems NEC

371	V999	PROBLEMS NEC IN CODES 008- TO V629
372	0994	(See after position number 23)
373	5997	(See after position number 173)
374	6254	(See after position number 188)
375	7900	(See after position number 298)
376	7950	(See after position numbers 298, 375, 51)
377	9952	(See after position number 334)
378	9950	(See after position number 337)

Appendix 2: An international glossary for primary care

Report of the Classification Committee of the World Organization of National Colleges, Academies and Academic Associations of General Practitioners/Family Physicians (WONCA).

Precise definitions of terms that describe the process of primary care are essential to the collection of primary health care data. Whenever possible, these definitions should be uniform and unambiguous. Research workers who wish to collaborate with or interpret work of colleagues from other countries can benefit from a standard glossary of commonly used health terms.

In response to these needs, the Classification Committee of the World Organization of National Colleges, Academies, and Academic Associations of General Practitioners/Family Physicians presents this document. Consensus on the definitions was reached by the Committee with consultation from general practice/family physician organizations and individuals. Existing primary care glossaries from several countries and the World Health Organization were also consulted.

The definitions provided are intended as guidelines, rather than absolute dicta, for primary care providers and researchers who desire comparability. New knowledge, drifts in use of language with time, and new processes will inevitably require revision of definitions and the addition of new terms. A comprehensive dictionary is not intended, but rather terms most commonly used are included.

Equivalent terms are enclosed in parentheses with the country of origin bracketed. It should be understood, however, that exact equivalence may not be present. It was not always possible to include fine shades of differences of meaning. For convenience, the male pronouns have been used throughout.

I. General

A. Health—A state of optimal physical, mental, and social well-being, and not merely the absence of disease or infirmity (modified World Health Organization definition).

B. Health care—Assessment, health maintenance, therapy, education, promotion of health, prevention of illness, and related activities (provided by qualified professionals) to improve or maintain health status.

C. Health care system—The organizational structure through which health care is provided.

D. Primary care* (Primary health care)—Primary health care is essential health care made universally accessible to individuals and families in the community by means acceptable to them, through their full participation and at a cost that the community and country can afford. It forms an integral part both of the country's health system of which it is the nucleus and of the overall social and economic development of the community (WHO–Alma Ata 1978). With regards to the work of general practitioners/family physicians this emphasizes responsibility for the patient beginning at the time of the first encounter and continuing thereafter. This includes overall management and co-ordination of health care, such as appropriate use of consultants, specialists, and other medical/health care resources. In addition, maintenance of continuity on a long-term basis, including co-ordination of secondary and tertiary is required.

E. Recorder—The person who records or supervises the recording of information under study.

F. Practice register—The list of all registered patients in a practice. See section IV-B-1 for the definition of a registered patient.

G. Age–sex register—The list of all registered patients by age and sex. The primary purpose of this register is to provide a defined population against which rates of observed occurrence of phenomena in a practice may be calculated. It can also be used to monitor immunization programs, identify groups at special risk, monitor practice size, plan physician education priorities, and for other purposes.

H. Diagnostic index (morbidity index, problem index, E book)—A system in which the diseases, illnesses, and social problems in a patient population are recorded by diagnosis or problem, date of presentation, patient name, age, and sex. This index helps in retrieval of medical records for cohorts of patients with similar health problems, and may be used to facilitate follow-up.

II. Provider descriptors

A. Health care provider—A qualified person who renders health care services.

1. Family physician/general practitioner. A physician who provides and co-ordinates personal, primary, and continuing comprehensive health care to individuals and families. He provides care for both sexes of all ages, for physical, behavioral, and social problems.

*This definition is a change from the original version.

2. Physician of first contact. The first physician seen by a patient during an episode of illness or injury, or for preventive and/or health-education matters.

3. Primary physician (primary care physician)—A family physician, general practitioner or other specialist who practises primary care.

4. Community physician—The primary concern of the community physician is the health status of the population within a defined geographical area. He is usually responsible for assessment and evaluation of the community's health needs and for the organization of health services to meet those needs. He will generally not render primary health care, except for specific disease entities such as selected communicable diseases. The role of a community physician varies from country to country, but he is usually employed by a government agency.

5. Locum tenens. A practitioner employed for a stated period of time by a physician to assume responsibility for the care of his practice population during an absence. Responsibility reverts to the principal physician upon his return.

6. Specialist. A physician with special competence and approved training in a particular field of medicine.

7. Consultant. A physician with special competence in a particular area of medicine who provides services related to this area at the request of another health care provider.

8. District physician. A primary physician who accepts continuing responsibility for the general health care of all persons living in a defined geographical area. In addition to his function as a general practitioner/ family physician, he often functions as a community physician, and is usually employed by a government agency either on a full- or part-time basis.

9. Physician in training (trainee assistant/trainee/assistant). The terms undergraduate, graduate, post-graduate, vocational, and continuing medical education have different meanings in different countries and at times are used inconsistently within a single country. The *table* on page 160 approximates common usages.

10. Ancillary staff. Non-medical personnel working in a practice, including nurse or practice sister, health visitor, medical social worker, secretary, practice aide, receptionist, administrator, business manager, book-keeper, and others. The ancillary staff differs from practice to practice, and from country to country.

11. Other health care providers. Qualified graduates (professionals and paraprofessionals) of disciplines other than medicine who also render health care. These include, for example, dentist, pharmacist, physician associate, medex physiotherapist, nurse-practitioner, graduate nurse, public health nurse, psychologist, social worker, minister of religion, and others. (The Committee invites these provider groups to submit definitions which describe their discipline.)

Table. Physicians in training

Training level	North America	United Kingdom, New Zealand, Australia, South Africa	Continental Europe
I. Basic sciences	Undergraduate	Undergraduate	Undergraduate
II. Medical school	Graduate	Undergraduate	Undergraduate
III. Initial post-medical school training	Internship (also used in Australia)	Pre-registration (houseman, junior intern)	Pre-license or post-graduate
IV. Specialization	Residency	Vocational	Graduate
V. Life long education	Continuing	Continuing	Post-graduate continuing

B. Health care team—A group of health care providers, who may represent several disciplines, and ancillary staff, working co-operatively to provide health care.

III. Practice descriptors

Practice. The organizational structure in which one or more physicians provide and supervise health care for a population of patients.

A. Manpower classification of practice

1. Solo practice (single-handed). A practice in which a single physician provides and supervises health care for a population of patients.

2. Group practice (co-operative practice [Denmark]). A practice in which the patient population is cared for by a number of associated/affiliated physicians. The principal responsibility for sub-groups of the population may be assigned to one or more physicians, but the group accepts the responsibility for continuity of patient care. In a legal sense, however, the individual physician usually has the ultimate responsibility for each patient.

(a) Single-specialty group—A group practice in which all physician members belong to the same specialty.

(b) Multi-specialty group—A group practice in which the physician members belong to more than one specialty.

3. Association of practices (group practice [Netherlands]). Practices of physicians who share premises, but not patients.

B. Geographical classification of practice populations—European recommendations for the 1970 population censuses (United Nations Publication No. ST/CES.13 1969) suggest that a distinction be made between urban, semi-urban, and rural areas. 'Since conditions vary considerably between countries, it is recognized that countries should be given latitude in selecting dividing lines between the three categories that are appropriate to their own conditions. However, in the interest of international comparability, countries should endeavor to select limits that approximate as closely as possible to 2000 and 10000. The definitions and limits should be clearly stated in the census report.' For the purposes of this glossary, the precise populations used to define urban, semi-urban, and rural areas were chosen arbitrarily. It is recognized that physicians within the various countries using this glossary may have different requirements. It is recommended that physicians who define geographical configurations of different population sizes state the numerical range they have chosen to define a geographical area.

1. Urban practice population. A practice serving a population, a majority of which are located in a city with a population of 50000 or more (20000 in New Zealand). For countries with a smaller population, a figure of 10000 may be used, but it should be specified. The designation *Metropolitan population* may be used for a conurbation with a population of 250000 or more.

2. Semi-urban practice population. A practice serving a population, a majority of which is located in a city with a population between 2000 and 50000. For countries with smaller populations, the range shall be between 2000 and 10000 population.

3. Rural practice population. A practice serving a discrete population, a majority of which is located in a town or scattered dwellings of less than 2000 population.

4. Other. Additional geographical population descriptors, such as *central city population, suburban population,* and *primitive or remote practice population* may be used, but the population size should be specifically defined in each case.

C. Practice sites

(a) Private office (surgery or surgery rooms [UK], consulting rooms [New Zealand], consulting rooms or surgery [South Africa])—The premises in which a physician conducts his practice. More than one practitioner and paramedical services may be accommodated in these premises.

(b) Residential office (residential surgery rooms [New Zealand and UK])—An office (surgery) which is located in a physician's home.

(c) Satellite office (satellite or branch surgery [UK], satellite rooms [New Zealand], suburban surgery [South Africa])—An office (surgery) located at a distance from the main site, office (surgery) or health centre. Staffing and the provision of health services is the responsibility of administration of the primary site.

(d) Health centre—A centre which emphasizes both total medical care and preventive personal health services. Staffing is varied and may include a group of family physicians/general practitioners, a multidisciplinary team, ancillary staff, specialists, and other health care providers. The centre may be owned by private physicians, government, or public agencies.

(e) Polyclinic. The definition of polyclinic varies in different countries. Usually it is a clinic attached to a hospital, with a medical staff largely comprised of specialists, often working independently, rather than as a team.

(f) Day hospital—A health care facility, providing day health care and monitoring facilities, with full medical and paramedical services available.

D. Mechanisms for reimbursement

1. Fee for service (private fees). A fee is assessed for each service or patient contact provided. Reimbursement may be from the patient and/or a third party.

2. Prepayment. The physician receives advance payment to provide specified health services for a particular patient or group of patients during a specified time period.

3. Capitation (allowances). A form of payment based on the number of registered patients, usually covering the full range of medical services provided.

4. Government sponsored/subsidized. Participating physicians receive reimbursement directly or indirectly from the government for services rendered to that portion of the population covered by the government plan. State insurance programs include Medicare in North America and the National Health Service in the United Kingdom.

5. Salary. The physician is an employee and receives a fixed wage for rendering medical care.

E. Special function practices

1. Teaching practice (training practice). A practice in which students (residents/registrars and medical students) are taught as an integral part of the practice.

2. Industrial practice. A practice conducted within the confines of an industrial organization. Usually the physician is reimbursed by salary, or according to the terms of a specific contract. Ancillary staff are usually employees of the industry.

3. Hospital practice. A practice conducted within the confines of a hospital. The source of patients, method of reimbursement, and relationships with ancillary staff are extremely variable, and should be defined for each specific instance.

4. Research practice. A practice organized and equipped for data collection and research studies.

F. Characteristics of practices

1. Appointment system. The system used by a physician to plan and regulate the timing of patient encounters. It may be *complete,* where no patients other than emergencies are seen except by appointment, or *partial,* where there is greater flexibility.

2. Clinic or special sessions. Occasions when patients of a similar type, or those suffering from the same condition, are grouped together for supervision, examination, treatment, discussion, or advice. Appointments may or may not be required. The type of clinic should be specified, e.g. *obstetric clinic* for antenatal and postnatal care; *child health clinic* for care of children and babies; *special clinics* for obesity, geriatrics, diabetes, and other conditions.

The use of the word clinic varies from country to country. In Australia 'special sessions' are held and the term clinic is reserved for group practices and/or their premises. In North America the term clinic may also mean a charitably operated practice or session. In Norway the term can mean either a little hospital or an out-patient department.

IV. Patient descriptors

Physicians who do not have registered or assigned lists of patients and families may require different definitions of the following terms, some of which are based on attendance frequencies in order to facilitate calculations of practice populations. In some countries (i.e. United Kingdom, the Netherlands, or Denmark) the registered lists often reflect the patient population with acceptable accuracy. In other countries (i.e. North America, Australia, or Norway) populations can only be estimated from utilization patterns.

Family. A group of persons sharing a common household. A relationship (including, but not necessarily limited by, blood or marriage ties) is implied. For purposes of this definition, persons who temporarily reside away from the household are included.

Household. Either (a) *one person household,* i.e. a person living alone in a separate room, suite of rooms, or housing unit; (b) a *multiperson household,* i.e. a group of two or more persons who combine to occupy the whole or part of a housing unit. The group may pool their incomes to a greater or lesser extent. The group may be composed of a family or of unrelated persons, or both, including *boarders* and excluding *lodgers.*

A. Family

1. Registered family. A family containing two or more members who receive health care from a practice.

2. Active registered family. Registered family containing at least one member who has received health care at least once in the past two years.

3. Attending family. A registered family containing at least one member who has received health care in the past year.

4. Inactive registered family. A registered family in which no member has received health care in the past two years.

5. Formerly registered family. A previously registered family which is no longer considered (by the practice or by personal determination) to be part of the practice population, and is removed from the register.

B. Patient—A person who receives or contracts for professional advice or services from a health care provider.

1. Registered patient. A patient who receives ongoing health care from a practice (excludes former, temporary, transient patients).

2. Visiting patient. A registered patient who has received services from the practice at least one time in the last two years. This includes attending patients.

3. Attending patient. A registered patient who has personally received services from the practice in the past year.

4. Nonvisiting patient. A registered patient who has received no services from the practice within the last two years.

5. Temporary or transient patient. A patient who receives one or more services from a practice, but who usually receives health care elsewhere.

6. Formerly registered patient. A patient (excluding temporary or transient) who has previously been registered, but who is no longer considered (by the practice or by personal determination) to be part of the practice population, and is removed from the register.

7. For practices registered by families

(a) Active registered patient—A registered patient who has received services from a practice at least once and belongs to a family, one member of which has received services within the last two years.

(b) Inactive registered patient—A registered patient who has received services from the practice at least once, but neither he nor any member of his family has received services within the last two years.

C. Statistics and analysis—The collection of the following demographic data is desirable:

1. Patient identification. Should be unique.

2. Residence. There are several options for the classification of residence which include address, telephone exchange, census tract, postal or zip code, grid, or municipal jurisdiction.

3. Date of birth. Should be collected in such a way that age may be calculated to the nearest year.

4. Sex of patient. Male or female.

5. Marital status. Married (includes common-law), single, separated, divorced, or widowed.

6. Ethnic origin. Black, white, other (patient determined).

7. Socioeconomic status. May be derived by several techniques which use occupation, education, income, method of payment, area of residence within census tracts, or a combination of two or more of these parameters.

V. Population descriptors

A. Practice population—The total number of active registered patients in a practice.

B. Study population—All patients included in a study during the period of a project.

C. Registered population—The total number of active registered patients in a practice, taken at the midpoint of a study. It is often difficult to count this population with precision. It may be possible to calculate the population from encounter data; if this is done, the method used should be specified.

D. Standard age groups—Less than 1; 1 to 4; 5 to 14; 15 to 24; 25 to 44; 45 to 64; 65 and greater. These groups may be subdivided into smaller cohorts (for example, 5 to 9 years) provided the standard division points are retained.

E. Patients at risk—Patients from the practice population considered to be at greater risk for a disease than other individuals in the same population.

F. Population at risk—A population of persons, with a geographically defined area, a random sample or a group selected for specific criteria from the greater population may be used. At times the registered patient population may be considered the population at risk.

VI. Morbidity descriptors

A. Problem—A provider-determined assessment of anything that concerns a patient, the provider (in relation to the health or the patient), or both. Problems should be recorded at the highest level of specificity determined at the time of that particular visit. The *International Classification of Health Problems in Primary Care* (*ICHPPC-2*) should be used to classify and code problems.

1. New problem. The first presentation of a problem, including the first presentation of a recurrence of a previously resolved problem, but excluding the presentation of a previously assessed problem to a different provider.

2. Continuing problem. A previously assessed problem which requires ongoing care. It includes follow-up for a problem or an initial presentation to a provider of a problem previously assessed by another provider.

B. Episode (attack, bout)—A problem or illness in a patient, over the entire period of time from its onset to its resolution.

C. Diagnosis—The formal statement of the provider's understanding of the patient's problem.

1. Principal diagnosis (main diagnosis). The most important problem, as determined by the health care provider. This should be coded to *ICHPPC-2*.

2. Associated diagnosis (concurrent diagnosis, sub-diagnosis). Another diagnosis made at the same time as the principal diagnosis.

3. Diagnostic criteria. Those signs, symptoms, and investigative findings that are essential to making a diagnosis.

D. Disease—The failure of the adaptive mechanisms of an organism to counteract adequately the stimuli or stresses to which it is subject, resulting in a disturbance in the function or structure of any part, organ, or system of that body.

1. Acute disease (short-term disease). An episode of disease with a duration of four weeks or less.

2. Subacute disease. An episode of disease with a duration of between four weeks and six months.

3. Chronic disease (long-term disease). An episode of disease with a duration of six months or more.

E. Illness—The patient's subjective perception of the disease process.

F. Impairment—Any reduction of functional, psychological, physiological, or anatomical capacity to participate in activities of daily living.

1. Temporary impairment. Impairment with an expected complete recovery.

2. Permanent impairment. Impairment in which a complete recovery is not expected.

G. Disability—Any restriction or lack (resulting from impairment) of ability to perform an activity in the manner or within the range, considered normal for a human being.

H. Handicap—A disadvantage for a given individual, resulting from an impairment or a disability, that limits or prevents the fulfilment of a role that is normal (depending on age, sex, and social and cultural factors) for that individual.

VII. Encounter descriptors

A. Encounter—Any professional interchange between a patient and one or more members of a health care team. One or more problems or diagnoses may be identified at each encounter. Analyses of encounter data should distinguish encounters from problems.

1. Direct encounter (face-to-face meeting). An encounter in which there is face-to-face meeting of a patient and professional.

(a) Office encounter (surgery encounter, attendance, consultation [UK and South Africa])—A direct encounter in the provider's office or surgery.

(b) Home encounter (housecall, visit [UK and Australia], home visit or housecall [South Africa])—A direct encounter occurring at the patient's residence (this includes home or a friend where a patient is visiting, hotel, room, etc.).

(c) Hospital encounter—A direct encounter in the hospital setting. One encounter is counted for each patient visit.

(1) Hospital in-patient encounter—A direct encounter with an in-patient.

(2) Out-patient encounter—A direct encounter with an out-patient in either the emergency room or the out-patient clinic.

(d) Problem contact—A patient provider transaction in regard to one problem. There may be several problem contacts during each encounter.

2. Indirect encounter. An encounter in which there is no physical or face-to-face meeting between the patient and the professional. These encounters may be subdivided by the mode of communication, e.g. *telephone encounter, written encounter,* or *encounter by message or through a third party.*

B. Referral—A referral is made when resources outside of any health care provider's command (whether in or outside of the practice) are requested on the patient's behalf. Patients may be referred for a specific service, a general opinion, or for other desirable reasons.

C. Consultation—In the United Kingdom, Australia, and New Zealand a consultation is an occasion on which a patient receives professional advice, help, or treatment at the doctor's premises. A domicilary consultation occurs when the doctor and a consultant meet at the patient's house to assess the patient. In North America a consultation is an exchange of information between doctors about a patient. The consultation may be informal (corridor consultation) or may involve the examination of the patient by the consultant in a more formal fashion, either in the presence of the primary care physician or in his absence, with a later exchange of information by verbal or written communication.

D. Time of encounter—The time at which the encounter occurs.

1. Encounter during scheduled hours. Encounters which occur during usual or posted working hours of the health care providers. These hours should be clearly stated.

2. Encounter during unscheduled hours. Encounters which occur at times other than the usual working hours of the health care providers, but which exclude night encounters. These hours should be clearly stated.

3. Night encounters. Encounters made betweem the hours of 2300 and 0700. If other time periods are chosen, these should be indicated.

E. Duration of encounter—The segment of time occupied by a single patient encounter.

VIII. Service descriptors

Service. An action taken by the provider in order to improve or maintain the health and well-being of the patient and/or the family.

A. Diagnostic (investigative) service. The assessment of any problem by history, physical examination, laboratory, X-ray, or other examinations performed either inside or outside of the office setting.

1. General assessment. A full history and detailed examination of those factors which determine the physical, mental, and social well-being of the patient with appropriate investigations, including a complete record of findings and advice for the patient.

2. Specific assessment. Includes a full history and detailed examination which relates to a specific diagnosis or problem with appropriate investigations, and including a complete record of findings, and advice for the patient.

B. Therapeutic services. These include pharmacological therapy, surgical therapy, physical therapy, psychotherapy, and others.

1. Supportive care. Services which promote the maintenance of bodily functions, but are generally not considered to be curative.

2. Emergency call service (deputizing service-emergency roster [Australia]). A service which provides temporary medical care for patients whose primary physician is off duty or absent from his practice.

3. Rehabilitation service. A service which promotes restoration of activities and social functioning following illness or injury, as nearly as possible to the premorbid level.

C. Preventive service. These include immunizations, screening tests, risk assessment, education, pre- and post-natal check-ups, well baby care, family planning, and other services.

1. Maternity services/care. Comprises the diagnosis of pregnancy, antenatal care, delivery, and post-natal care, including a final follow-up examination.

2. Newborn care. Routine care of the well baby, including all visits and necessary instructions to the mother. The time period used to designate this care should be specified. The *perinatal period* includes the first 7 days following birth, while the *neonatal period* includes the first 28 days after birth.

3. Well baby care. Periodic office encounters with well babies during the first two years of life, for routine supervision, assessment of growth and development, and any required parental instructions. These would include measurements and immunizations as necessary.

4. Premature baby care. All hospital encounters with premature babies with a birth-weight of less than 5½ pounds or 2.5 kilograms.

5. Primary prevention. Measures designed to reduce the incidence of disease in an individual or a population by reducing the risk of onset, prevention of occurrence, and control of spread.

6. Secondary prevention. Measures designed to reduce the effect and prevalence of disease in an individual or population by shortening its course and duration.

7. Tertiary prevention. Measures designed to reduce the effect and prevalence of a chronic disability in an individual or a population by minimizing the functional impairment consequent to the disease or accident.

8. Screening. The attempt to identify unrecognized disease or defect in an individual or population by means of tests and/or other methods which discriminate between those who probably have or are at risk for a given disease and those who are not so affected.

9. Health promotion. Services designed to help the patient avoid illness and maintain good health.

D. Administrative services—Services which derive from the responsible position accorded to health care providers by the community, e.g. witnessing of signatures, attestations about character, certifying fitness for certain functions (driving, work, sports), and unfitness for certain functions.

E. Community care—The care and supervision of persons outside the hospital by medical and social agencies that are based in the community.

IX. Standard reporting

Rates. Rates are defined as the number of events occurring in a study population in a given period of time, divided by the size of the study population. According to previous definitions, a study population may be made up of any of the following groups: registered patients, active patients, inactive patients, etc. Rates per hundred or per thousand are typical, but this may change to per 10000 or per 100000 as the frequency of the event decreases. For some rates the study population of patients may not constitute the denominator, which instead may refer to the provider, e.g. the number of patients seen per week per provider. Thus, we may construct rates with one of the following numerators: problems, encounters or services, patients, families, etc., and one of the following denominators: provider, team, practice, study population, registered patient population, census population, random sample population, etc.

Adjusted rates. Two practices may generate different rates for reasons unconnected with the underlying morbidity or operation of a practice. Thus, the direct encounter rate per 100 patients in an active patient population will vary according to the age and sex composition of that population. To compare crude rates between practices, it may be necessary to standardize them by age and sex. The 'adjusted rates' become comparable in spite of age and sex differences of the study population.

A. Encounter rates—Encounter rates may be tabulated using various numerators and denominators and it is important to define clearly the content of each. Thus, for numerators, direct encounters must be distinguished from indirect encounters, first encounters from repeat encounters, active patients from inactive patients, etc. For denominators, the method used to define the practice population should be specified. The following rates are examples chosen from numerous possible encounter rates.

1. Patient encounter rate. The number of patients who attend during the survey (counting each patient only once), divided by the practice population at the mid-point of the survey.

2. Work load rate. The number of encounters (direct, face-to-face) during the survey, divided by the practice population at the midpoint of the survey.

3. Late encounter rate. The number of visits out of scheduled hours may be tabulated in several ways. For example:

(a) Per 1000 active registered patients.

(b) Per 100 direct patient encounters.

(c) Per 100 patients attending (counting each patient only once).

4. Hospitalization or referral rates. The number of patients hospitalizations or referrals during the survey, divided by the practice population at the mid-point of the survey.

B. Morbidity–mortality rates, incidence and prevalence. As with encounter rates, the content of both the numerator and the denominator must be specified.

1. Episode of illness rate. An episode of illness may be hard (indeed impossible) to define; for example, it is difficult to know when an episode of peptic ulcer in an individual starts and ends (i.e. did it heal and reactivate, or did it continue without symptoms), but this can be circumvented for most such conditions by counting each single diagnosis as an episode, however often during the survey that patient may visit for it. Thus, if a patient with a peptic ulcer visits his doctor on one or more occasions during the survey for this condition, it is counted as a single episode, however far apart in time the encounters may be. For conditions, such as injuries, it is usually simple to differentiate one episode from another. Usually episodes of illness are recorded by diagnosis so one may calculate the number of episodes of a given illness per 1000 patients in a practice population.

2. Mortality rate (crude death rate). The number of deaths that occur among a population during a year, divided by the average number of persons 'at risk' during the same year (expressed per 1000 persons).

3. Fatality rate. The number of deaths from a disease recorded during a defined period, divided by the total number of cases of that disease recorded during the same period (expressed per 100 cases per year).

4. Incidence. The number of new cases of a given disease arising within a defined population during a defined period of time.

5. Prevalence. The number of cases of a given disease present in a defined population at one point in time (point prevalence) or during a defined period of time (period prevalence).

Acknowledgement

This publication was supported in part by NIH Grant LM03289 from the National Library of Medicine and Rockefeller Foundation Grant # GAHS 8037.

This report prepared by WONCA does not necessarily represent primary health care terminology by WHO.

Alphabetical index

The ICHPPC alphabetical index does not contain all of the variations and synonyms of terms found in the tabular section which should be consulted as the primary coding instrument. It does, however, contain several diagnostic titles which are not found in the tabular section. For terms not listed in this index, the recorder is advised to consult volume 2, Alphabetical Index of the *International Classification of Diseases*, ninth Revision (*ICD-9*).

As with the index of *ICD-9* this section is organized in the form of lead terms (main entries) at the left of the column, with various levels of indentation that identify the variations or anatomical sites. Usually the lead term is the name of the disease or health problem. For the supplementary section, Chapter XVIII, key words such as 'counseling' and 'examination' are the main entries.

The code numbers found in the alphabetical index are those assigned to *ICHPPC-2*. Equivalent *ICD-9* code numbers may be obtained by consulting the tabular section. Abbreviations are the same as those listed in the introduction. Parentheses are used to enclose synonyms or explanatory phrases that may or may not be present in the diagnostic title. Spelling is consistent with United States convention. Familiarity with the contents of the tabular section will make this alphabetical index more useful.

Each entry in the index is followed by three numbers:
(1) page number of tabular list;
(2) position number in tabular list;
(3) ICHPPC code.

Abdomen, abdominal
acute 112, *279*, **7890**
pain 112, *279*, **7890**
Abnormal, abnormalities (of)
bone development 106, *252*, **758-**
cholesterol levels 44, *56*, **272-**
electrocardiogram tracing 115, *229*, **793-**
excitability under minor stress 51, *71*, **3001**
gait 115, *300*, **7889**
hematocrit or hemoglobin 114, *(375)*, **7900**
increase in development 115, *300*, **7889**
lipoprotein levels 44, *56*, **272-**
menstrual periods, NOS 89, *193*, **6269**
pap smear 115, *(376)*, **7950**
platelets 46, *62*, **287-**
pregnancy—*see* Pregnancy
red cells 114, *(375)*, **7900**
results, unexplained,
        of investigations NEC 115, *299*, **793-**
teeth, dentition or formation 76, *148*, **520-**
test findings, NEC 115, *299*, **793-**
        biochemical 114, *(51)*, **7902**
        blood chemistry 114, *(51)*, **7902**
        coagulation tests 46, *62*, **287-**
ECG 115, *299*, **793-**
function studies 115, *299*, **793-**
glucose tolerance, not
        yet diagnosed 115, *(51)*, **7902**
serology 115, *299,* **793-**
SMA 114, *(51)*, **7902**
X-ray not yet diagnosed 115, *299*, **793-**
triglycerides level 44, *56*, **272-**
white cells 46, *64*, **288-**
Abortion 93, *201*, **634-**
advice on 126, *354*, **V654**
history of habitual (currently pregnant)
        93, *202*, **648-**
        without current pregnancy 89, *194*, **629-**
incomplete 93, *201*, **634-**
induced 92, *200*, **636-**
        with complications 92, *200*, **636-**
missed 93, *201*, **634-**
spontaneous 93, *201*, **634-**
threatened 91, *197*, **640-**
Abrasion (corneal) (skin) 121, *326*, **918-**
infected 121, *333*, **959-**
Abscess
abdominal 95, *207*, **680-**
accessory sinus 70, *134*, **461-**
amebic 31, *1*, **008-**
ankle 95, *207*, **680-**
anorectal 79, *162*, **565-**
antecubital space 95, *207*, **680-**
anus 79, *162*, **565-**
arm 95, *207*, **680-**
axilla 95, *207*, **680-**
Bartholin's gland 89, *194*, **629-**
breast 86, *182*, **611-**
        postpartum or puerperal 94, *206*, **670-**

Brodie's 105, *246*, **739-**
buccal cavity 76, *149*, **528-**
buttock 95, *207*, **680-**
cheek 95, *207*, **680-**
chin 95, *207*, **680-**
conjunctiva 57, *92*, **3720**
cul-de-sac 87, *183*, **614-**
dental 76, *148*, **520-**
ear 59, *101*, **3820**
eyelid 57, *93*, **3730**
face 95, *207*, **680-**
finger 95, *207*, **680-**
foot 95, *207*, **680-**
    toe 95, *207*, **680-**
genital organ
    female 89, *194*, **629-**
    male 86, *180*, **607-**
groin 95, *207*, **680-**
hand 95, *207*, **680-**
    finger 95, *207*, **680-**
ischiorectal 79, *162*, **565-**
jaw 76, *148*, **520-**
labium 89, *194*, **629-**
leg 95, *207*, **680-**
loin 95, *207*, **680-**
lung 75, *147*, **519-**
lymphatic gland or node 95, *209*, **683-**
    mesenteric 46, *63*, **2891**
mouth 76, *149*, **528-**
nose
    external 95, *207*, **680-**
    internal 75, *146*, **4781**
palmar space 95, *207*, **680-**
pararectal 79, *162*, **565-**
pelvis
    female 87, *183*, **614-**
    male 95, *207*, **680-**
perianal 79, *162*, **565-**
perirectal 79, *162*, **565-**
peritonsillar 70, *135*, **463-**
pharyngeal 75, *147*, **519-**
pilonidal 95, *211*, **685-**
pulmonary 75, *147*, **519-**
rectum 79, *162*, **565-**
salivary gland 76, *149*, **528-**
scrotum 86, *180*, **607-**
sebaceous 98, *220*, **7062**
site (other) 95, *207*, **680-**
skin 95, *207*, **680-**
stitch 122, *336*, **998-**
subcutaneous 95, *207*, **680-**
thumb 95, *207*, **680-**
toe 95, *207*, **680-**
tonsil 70, *135*, **463-**
vagina 87, *185*, **6161**
vulva 89, *194*, **629-**
Absence (of)
acquired
        extremities, any part 104, *245*, **736-**

Advice
family planning 126, *347*, **V256**
health instruction or education 126, *354*,
 V654
problems external to patient 127, *355*,
 V651
Aerophagia 51, *71*, **3001**
Aftercare
check-up, no disease 123, *338*, **V70-**
management of high-risk prosthetic
 device or implant 124, *342*, **V10-**
patient on high-risk medication 123, *341*,
 V14-
After-cataract 58, *96*, **366-**
Agalactia 94, *205*, **676-**
Agammaglobulinemia 44, *57*, **279-**
Agitation 55, *86*, **316-**
Agranulocytosis 46, *64*, **288-**
Albinism 44, *57*, **279-**
Albuminuria
arising during pregnancy 93, *202*, **648-**
orthostatic 84, *173*, **5936**
 NOS 114, *(357)*, **7900**
postural 84, *173*, **5936**
puerperal 93, *202*, **648-**
Alcoholism, alcoholic
acute intoxication 54, *80*, **3031**
addiction 54, *80*, **3031**
cardiopathy 54, *80*, **3031**
cirrhosis of liver 80, *165*, **571-**
delirium 54, *80*, **3031**
dementia 54, *80*, **3031**
gastritis, chronic 77, *153*, **536-**
hepatitis 80, *165*, **571-**
Aleukemia 39, *38*, **201**
Alkalosis 44, *57*, **279-**
Allergy, allergic NOS 122, *(378)*, **9950**
due to
 adhesive tape 97, *214*, **692-**
 airborne substance 74, *145*, **477-**
 animal dander or hair 74, *145*, **477-**
 beesting (anaphylactic shock) 120, *325*,
  910-
 cold weather 97, *214*, **692-**
 cosmetic 97, *214*, **692-**
 detergent 97, *214*, **692-**
 drug (any) (external) (internal) 122,
  (377), **9952**
  dermatitis 97, *214*, **692-**
  wrong substance or overdose 122, *334*,
   977-
 dust 74, *145*, **477-**
 dye 97, *214*, **692-**
 feathers 74, *145*, **477-**
 food 97, *214*, **692-**
  atopic 97, *214*, **692-**
 gastroenteritis or colitis 78, *159*, **558-**
 grass 74, *145*, **477-**
  asthmatic 74, *144*, **493-**

 heat or hot weather 97, *214*, **692-**
 inhalant 74, *145*, **477-**
 plant leaf contact 97, *214*, **692-**
 pollen (ragweed) 74, *145*, **477-**
  asthmatic 74, *144*, **493-**
 serum (anaphylactic shock) 122, *336*,
  998-
 solvent 97, *214*, **692-**
 tobacco 97, *214*, **692-**
 test 122, *(378)*, **9950**
Alopecia 98, *222*, **704-**
syphilitic 35, *22*, **090-**
Altitude, high, effect of 122, *337*, **994-**
Amaurosis fugax 58, *99*, **378-**
Amblyopia 38, *99*, **378-**
Ameba, amebic
carrier or suspected carrier 123, *339*,
 V01-
coli 31, *1*, **008-**
Amebiasis, any site 31, *1*, **008-**
Amenorrhea 89, *189*, **6260**
Amino-acid deficiency 44, *57*, **279-**
Amnesia, hysterical or psychogenic 51, *71*,
 3001
Amputation
stump, painful or with
 late complications 122, *336*, **998-**
traumatic, any limb(s) 120, *323*, **889-**
Amputee 104, *245*, **736-**
Amyloidosis 44, *57*, **279**
Anacidity, gastric 77, *153*, **536**
psychogenic 51, *71*, **3001**
Anaphylactic shock or reaction 122, *378*,
 9950
following bite or sting 120, *325*, **910-**
from
 medicines 122, *(378)*, **9950**
 nonmedicinal agents 122, *335*, **989-**
 serum or immunization 122, *336*,
  998-
Anemia NOS 46, *61*, **285-**
achlorhydric 45, *58*, **280-**
agranulocytic 46, *64*, **288-**
aplastic 46, *61*, **285-**
atypical 46, *61*, **285-**
combined system disease 45, *59*, **281-**
Cooley's 46, *60*, **282-**
deficiency NOS 45, *59*, **281-**
 folic acid 45, *59*, **281-**
 iron 45, *58*, **280-**
 of pregnancy 93, *202*, **468-**
due to blood loss 45, *58*, **280-**
during pregnancy 93, *202*, **648-**
hemolytic NOS 46, *60*, **282-**
 acquired 46, *61*, **285-**
 hereditary 46, *60*, **282-**
hyperchromic 45, *58*, **280-**
 of pregnancy 93, *202*, **468-**
iron deficiency 45, *58*, **280-**

Anemia (*cont.*)
macrocytic 45, *59*, **281-**
of pregnancy 93, *202*, **648-**
megaloblastic 45, *59*, **281-**
of pregnancy 93, *202*, **648-**
postpartum 93, *202*, **648-**
microcytic 45, *58*, **280-**
familial 46, *60*, **282-**
myeloblastic or myelocytic 39, *38*, **201-**
newborn 107, *253*, **778-**
posthemorrhagic 107, *253*, **778-**
normocytic NOS 46, *61*, **285-**
nutritional 45, *59*, **281-**
pernicious 45, *59*, **281-**
secondary 46, *61*, **285-**
sickle cell 46, *60*, **282-**
thrombocytopenic 46, *62*, **287-**
Anesthesia
sensation 109, *259*, **7820**
surgical assist 126, *353*, **V50-**
Aneurysm
abdominal 69, *132*, **459-**
aortic 69, *132*, **459-**
valve 64, (*111*), **424-**
carotid 69, *132*, **459-**
cerebrovascular (arteriosclerotic) 66, *124*,
438-
congenital 106, *247*, **746-**
heart 62, *110*, **412-**
acute 62, *109*, **412-**
site, other NEC 69, *132*, **459-**
valve 64, (*111*), **424-**
Angiectasis 69, *132*, **459-**
Angiitis 69, *132*, **459-**
Angina (pectoris) 62, *110*, **412-**
Ludwig's 76, *149*, **528-**
Vincent's 37, *31*, **136-**
Angioedema 122, (*378*), **9950**
Angiofibroma 41, *45*, **229-**
Angioma (benign) (cavernous) 41, *44*, **228-**
senile 69, *132*, **459-**
spider 69, *132*, **459-**
stellate 69, *132*, **459-**
Angiomatosis 106, *252*, **758-**
multiple sites 106, *252*, **758-**
Angioneurosis 51, *71*, **3001**
Angiospasm (traumatic) 67, *126*, **443-**
nerve 57, *91*, **355-**
Aniscoria 58, *99*, **378-**
Ankylosis, ankylosing
joint produced by surgical fusion 124, *342*,
V10-
sacroiliac 103, *241*, **7274**
spondylitis (spine) 100, *228*, **714-**
Anomaly
heart or circulatory structure 106, *247*,
746-
lower limb 106, *248*, **754-**
site, other NEC 106, *252*, **758-**

toenail 106, *252*, **758-**
Anorexia NOS 111, *273*, **7830**
hysterical 51, *71*, **3001**
nervosa 55, *86*, **316-**
Anosmia 115, *300*, **7889**
hysterical 51, *71*, **3001**
Anovulatory cycle 90, *195*, **606-**
Anthracosilicosis 75, *147*, **519-**
Anxiety (neurosis) (reaction) (state) 50, *70*,
3000
depression 52, *72*, **3004**
hysteria 52, *73*, **3009**
Aortic stenosis 64, (*111*), **424-**
Aphakia, acquired 58, *99*, **378-**
Aphasia 109, *257*, **7845**
Apnea 111, *269*, **7860**
Appendicitis 77, *154*, **540-**
Appetite
depraved or perverted 55, *86*, **316-**
excessive 115, *300*, **7889**
lack or loss of 111, *273*, **7830**
Arcus senilis 58, *99*, **378-**
Arrest, cardiac 64, *118*, **429-**
Arrhythmia NOS 64, *118*, **429-**
ectopic 63, *115*, **4276**
Arteriosclerosis or atherosclerosis
(arteriosclerotic) NOS 66, *125*, **440-**
cardiovascular 62, *110*, **412-**
cerebral (brain) 66, *124*, **438-**
cerebrovascular 66, *124*, **438-**
extremities 66, *125*, **440-**
generalized 66, *125*, **440-**
heart disease NOS 62, *110*, **412-**
valvular 64, (*111*), **424-**
obliterans 66, *124*, **438-**
occlusive 66, *124*, **438-**
pulmonary 64, *117*, **416-**
transient ischemic attack 66, *123*, **435-**
with hypertension, code also
hypertension
Arteritis NOS 69, *132*, **459-**
cerebral 66, *124*, **438-**
giant cell 69, *132*, **459-**
other NEC 69, *132*, **459-**
syphilitic 35, *22*, **090-**
Arthralgia 101, (*228*), **7194**
Arthritis 101, *231*, **725-**
acute, nonpyogenic or pyogenic 101, *231*,
725-
allergic 101, *231*, **725-**
atrophic 100, *228*, **714-**
chronic 101, *231*, **725-**
climacteric 101, *231*, **725-**
deformans 100, *229*, **715-**
spine 102, *237*, **721-**
degenerative 100, *229*, **715-**
spine 102, *237*, **721-**
due to Reiter's urethritis 37, *31*, **136-**
erythema epidemic 37, *31*, **136-**

Bigeminy rhythm 64, *118*, **429-**
Biliary dyskinesia 81, *166*, **574-**
Birthmark, NOS 106, *252*, **758-**
Bites
animal 120, *323*, **889-**
chigger 37, *30*, **133-**
insect 120, *325*, **910-**
poisonous
animal 122, *335*, **989-**
insect 120, *325*, **910-**
reptile 122, *335*, **989-**
snake 122, *335,* **989-**
venomous—*see* Bites, poisonous
Black eye due to contusion 121, *387*, **929-**
Blackhead 98, *224*, **7061**
Blackout 110, *264*, **7802**
Blast injury—*see* 120, *322*, **850-** to 121, *333*, **959-**
Blastomycosis 37, *31*, **136-**
Bleeding—*see also* Hemorrhage
ear 60, *107*, **388-**
eye 58, *99*, **378-**
during pregnancy 91, *197*, **640-**
gastrointestinal NOS 79, *276*, **578-**
gums 76, *148*, **520-**
intermenstrual 89, *193*, **6269**
oral 76, *149*, **528-**
per rectum 79, *164*, **5693**
postmenopausal 88, *187*, **627-**
stools 79, *276*, **578-**
stump 122, *336*, **998-**
umbilical 107, *253*, **778-**
uterine 89, *193*, **6269**
vaginal 89, *194*, **629-**
Blennorrhea 36, *23*, **098-**
inclusion 107, *253*, **778-**
Blepharitis (bacterial) (seborrhoeic) (staphylococcal) (ulcerative) 57, *93*, **3730**
Blepharospasm 57, *91*, **355-**
Blindness
acquired or congenital one or both eyes 58, *98*, **369-**
color 58, *99*, **378-**
due to refractive error 58, *94*, **367-**
night 58, *99*, **378-**
word 52, *74*, **315-**
Blister, skin 121, *326*, **918-**
Bloating 112, *278*, **7873**
Block, blocked
eustachian tube 59, *103*, **3815**
heart (A-V) 64, *118*, **429-**
tear duct 58, *99*, **378-**
congenital 106, *251*, **7436**
Blood donor 127, *355*, **V651**
potential, examination of 123, *338*, **V70-**
Bloody
discharge 115, *300*, **7889**
nose 111, *267*, **7847**

Bloodshot eyes 58, *99*, **378-**
Blue diaper syndrome 44, *57*, **279-**
Blurred vision 58, *99*, **378-**
Boil
auditory meatus, external 95, *207*, **680-**
axilla 95, *207*, **680-**
finger 95, *207*, **680-**
genital, male NEC 86, *180*, **607-**
groin 95, *207*, **680-**
nose
inside 75, *146*, **4781**
outside 95, *307*, **680-**
seminal vesicles 85, *176*, **601-**
site, other NEC 95, *207*, **680-**
toe 95, *207*, **680-**
Botulism 31, *1*, **008-**
Bowel discomfort 112, *279*, **7890**
Bowleg 104, *245*, **736-**
Bradycardia, sinus 64, *118*, **429-**
Breathing problem 111, *269*, **7860**
Bright's disease 82, *168*, **580-**
Brittle hair 98, *222*, **704-**
Broken blood vessel 68, *129*, **454-**
Bronchiectasis 74, *142*, **491-**
Bronchiolitis, acute 72, *138*, **466-**
Bronchitis,
acute 72, *138*, **466-**
asthmatic 74, *144*, **493-**
chronic 74, *142*, **491-**
fibrinous, acute 72, *138*, **466-**
NOS 72, *138*, **466-**
Bronchopneumonia 73, *140*, **486-**
Bronchospasm 75, *147*, **519-**
Brucellosis 37, *31*, **136-**
Bruise with intact skin 121, *327*, **929-**
Bruit 110, (*116*), **7852**
Bruxism 51, *71*, **3001**
Buerger's disease 67, *126*, **443-**
Bundle branch block 64, *118*, **429-**
Bunion (bunionette) 104, *245*, **736-**
Burn
chemical
external 121, *328*, **949-**
internal (ingestion) 121, *328*, **949-**
electric 121, *328*, **949-**
first, second, or third degree 121, *328*, **949-**
friction 121, *326*, **918-**
irradiation 121, *328*, **949-**
pressure 121, *326*, **918-**
sun 97, *214*, **692-**
Burning
eyes 58, *99*, **378-**
feet syndrome 43, *52*, **260-**
rectal 115, *300*, **7889**
sensation 109, *259*, **7820**
urination 112, *280*, **7881**
Bursitis NOS 102, *223*, **7263**
olecranon (elbow) 102, *223*, **7263**
popliteal 102, *223*, **7263**

Bursitis NOS (*cont.*)
prepatellar 102, *223*, **7263**
radiohumeral 102, *223*, **7263**
shoulder 101, *232*, **7260**
subacromial 101, *232*, **7260**

Cachexia 113, *293*, **7832**
Calcification, calcified
prostatic 86, *180*, **607-**
tendon 102, *233*, **7263**
Calculus
renal 83, *171*, **592**
staghorn 83, *171*, **592-**
urethral 83, *171*, **592-**
Callosity 98, *219*, **700-**
Cancer—*see* Neoplasm, malignant
Candidiasis, candidosis (mucosal)
cervix 36, *26*, **1121**
diaper 36, *26*, **1121**
oral cavity 36, *25*, **112-**
rectal 36, *25*, **113-**
site, other NEC 36, *25*, **112-**
urogenital 36, *26*, **1121**
vagina 36, *26*, **1121**
Canker (mouth) (sore) 76, *149*, **528-**
Capsulitis, adhesive, shoulder 101, *232*, **7260**
Carbuncle—*see* Boil
Carcinoma—*see also* Neoplasm,
malignant
in situ, cervix 39, *36*, **180-**
Cardiac dropsy 63, *112*, **428-**
Cardiomegaly 64, *118*, **429-**
Cardiomyopathy 64, *118*, **429-**
Cardiosclerosis 62, *110*, **412-**
Cardiospasm 76, *150*, **530-**
Caries, teeth 76, *148*, **520-**
Carotid
bruit 115, *300*, **7889**
plaque 66, *125*, **440-**
sinus syndrome 57, *91*, **355-**
Carotidynia 57, *91*, **355-**
Carpal tunnel syndrome 57, *91*, **355-**
Carrier (suspected) of parasitic
or infective disease 123, *339*, **V01-**
Caruncle—*see also* Boil
urethra 84, *174*, **598-**
Cataract, all types 58, *96*, **366-**
Catarrh of eustachian tube 59, *103*, **3815**
Catheter change 130, *371*, **V999**
Cat-scratch fever 37, *31*, **136-**
Cauda equina syndrome 57, *91*, **355-**
Cauliflower ear 105, *246*, **739-**
Causalgia syndrome 57, *91*, **355-**
Celiac disease, infantile or adult 81, *167*,
579-
Cellulitis
drainage site, postoperative 122, *366*, **998-**
ear, external 59, *100*, **3801**
ear lobe 95, *207*, **680-**

eyelid 57, *93*, **3730**
finger 95, *207*, **680-**
foot 95, *207*, **680-**
genital organ
gonococcal 36, *23*, **098-**
male 86, *180*, **607-**
hand 95, *207*, **680-**
lips 76, *149*, **528-**
mouth 76, *149*, **528-**
nose, inside 75, *147*, **519-**
orbital 58, *99*, **378-**
perirectal 79, *162*, **565-**
site, other NEC 95, *207*, **680-**
thumb 95, *207*, **680-**
toe 95, *207*, **680-**
Cephalgia, nonorganic 53, *76*, **3078**
Cephalhematoma
birth injury 107, *253*, **778-**
other 121, *327*, **929-**
Cerebrovascular disease 66, *124*, **438-**
Certificate completion 125, *348*, **V680-**
Cerumen 60, *106*, **3804**
Cervical
erosion 87, *184*, **622-**
rib syndrome 106, *252*, **758-**
root syndrome 102, *255*, **723-**
Cervicalgia 102, *235*, **723-**
Cervicitis 87, *184*, **622-**
Cervicobrachial syndrome 102, *235*, **723-**
Cestode infestation 37, *28*, **127-**
Chalazion 57, *93*, **3730**
Chancre 35, *22*, **090-**
Chancroid 37, *31*, **136-**
Change in bowel habits 81, *167*, **579-**
Chapping skin 99, *227*, **709-**
Charcot's joint 35, *22*, **090-**
nonvenereal 101, *231*, **725-**
Charley-horse, quadriceps 120, *321*, **848-**
Cheilitis 76, *149*, **528-**
Cheilosis angular 76, *149*, **528-**
Chemotherapy
maintenance 130, *371*, **V999**
prophylactic NEC 123, *339*, **V01-**
Chest-wall syndrome 110, *262*, **7865**
Chiari–Frommel syndrome 94, *205*, **676-**
Chickenpox 32, *9*, **052-**
Chigger bite 37, *30*, **133-**
Chilblains 122, *337*, **994-**
Chills 115, *300*, **7889**
Chloasma 92, *227*, **709-**
Choking 115, *300*, **7889**
Cholangitis 81, *166*, **574-**
Cholecystitis 81, *166*, **574-**
Cholecystolithiasis 81, *166*, **574-**
Choledocholithiasis 81, *166*, **574-**
Cholelithiasis 81, *166*, **574-**
Cholesteatoma 60, *107*, **388-**
Chondrocalcinosis, articular 44, *57*, **279-**
Chondrodysplasia 106, *252*, **758-**

Contraction, contracture (*cont.*)
pelvis 105, *246*, **739-**
plantar fascia 102, *234*, **728-**
premature heartbeat 63, *115*, **4276**
scar, skin 99, *227*, **709-**
socket, eye 58, *99*, **378-**
spine 103, *240*, **737-**
tendon (sheath) 102, *223*, **7263**
toe 104, *245*, **736-**
urethral orifice 84, *174*, **598-**
vaginal outlet 89, *194*, **629-**
vesical (neck) 84, *174*, **598-**
Volkmann's (ischemic) 121, *333*, **959-**
Contusion
eye 121, *327*, **929-**
with intact skin surface 121, *327*, **929-**
Conversion
hysteria, any type 51, *71*, **3001**
reaction (neurosis) 51, *71*, **3001**
tuberculous 31, *4*, **011-**
Convulsions 109, *254*, **7803**
febrile 109, *254*, **7803**
newborn 107, *253*, **778-**
COPD 74, *143*, **492-**
Cor pulmonale 64, *117*, **416-**
Corn 98, *219*, **700-**
Corneal abrasion 121, *326*, **918-**
Coronary
sinus rhythm 64, *118*, **429-**
thrombosis or infarction 62, *109*, **410-**
healed 62, *110*, **412-**
Coryza 70, *133*, **460-**
Costochondritis 105, *246*, **739-**
Cough 111, *270*, **7862**
Counseling NEC 130, *371*, **V999**
Cowpox 37, *31*, **136-**
Coxa valgus 104, *245*, **736-**
Coxsackie
infection (virus) NOS 37, *31*, **136-**
specified disease 37, *31*, **136-**
Cramps
abdomen 112, *279*, **7890**
legs 102, (*286*), **7295**
muscle 102, (*286*), **7295**
Craniostosis 106, *252*, **758-**
Creeping eruption 37, *28*, **127-**
Cretinism 42, *49*, **244-**
Crohn's disease 79, *160*, **555-**
Croup 17, *137*, **464-**
asthmatic 74, *144*, **493-**
bronchial 72, *138*, **466-**
diphtheritic 37, *31*, **136-**
false 75, *147*, **519-**
Crush
syndrome 121, *333*, **959-**
with
dislocation—*see* Dislocation
fracture—*see* Fracture
intact skin surface 121, *327*, **929-**

internal organ injury 121, *333*, **959-**
nerve injury 121, *333*, **959-**
open wound—*see* Wound, open
Cryptitis 79, *163*, **5646**
Cryptorchism 106, *249*, **7525**
Crypt tonsil 70, *135*, **463-**
Curvature of spine NOS 103, *240*, **737-**
Cushingoid 122, *334*, **977-**
correct substance, properly
administered 44, *57*, **279-**
Cushing's syndrome 44, *57*, **279-**
Cut—*see* Wound, open
Cyanosis 115, *300*, **7889**
Cyclothymic personality 54, *84*, **301-**
Cyst
Baker's 102, *233*, **7263**
Bartholin's 89, *194*, **629-**
breast, benign 86, *181*, **610-**
bronchial 75, *147*, **519-**
cerebellum 57, *91*, **355-**
cervix uteri 89, *194*, **629-**
ear 98, *220*, **7062**
epidermoid 98, *220*, **7062**
mouth or oral soft tissue 76, *149*, **528-**
epithelial 98, *220*, **7062**
eye 58, *99*, **378-**
follicular 89, *194*, **629-**
implantation dermoid 99, *227*, **709-**
iris 58, *99*, **378-**
mouth 76, *149*, **528-**
vagina or vulva 89, *194*, **629-**
inclusion dermoid 98, *220*, **7062**
kidney 106, *252*, **758-**
knee (semilunar cartilage) 104, *244*, **717-**
lip 76, *149*, **528-**
Meibomian, infected 57, *93*, **3730**
ovary 89, *194*, **629-**
penis 86, *180*, **607-**
periodontal 76, *148*, **520-**
pilonidal 95, *211*, **685-**
popliteal 106, *252*, **758-**
rectal 81, *167*, **579-**
renal 106, *252*, **758-**
sebaceous 98, *220*, **7062**
synovial 102, *233*, **7263**
thyroglossal duct 106, *252*, **758-**
vaginal 89, *104*, **629-**
Cystic
disease of breast, chronic 86, *181*, **610-**
fibrosis 44, *57*, **279-**
arising during pregnancy
or puerperium 91, *198*, **6466**
Cystocele 88, *186*, **618-**
Cystostomy 124, *342*, **V10-**
Cytology examination 123, *338*, **V70-**

Dacryocystitis 58, *99*, **378-**
Dandruff 96, *212*, **690-**
Darier's disease 106, *252*, **758-**

Deformity, nose *(cont.)*
  congenital 106, *252*, **758-**
  septum 75, *147*, **519-**
pelvis
  acquired 105, *246*, **739-**
  congenital 106, *252*, **758-**
saddle nose 105, *246*, **739-**
shoulder
  acquired 104, *245*, **736-**
    abduction, adduction,
      contraction, extension,
      flexion, or rotation 105, *246*, **739-**
  congenital 106, *252*, **758-**
spine
  acquired 105, *246*, **739-**
  congenital 106, *252*, **758-**
  kyphotic 103, *240*, **737-**
  rachitic 43, *52*, **260-**
  scoliotic 103, *240,* **737-**
thigh, acquired 104, *245*, **736-**
thumb, acquired 104, *245*, **736-**
wrist
  acquired 104, *245*, **736-**
    abduction, adduction,
      contraction, extension,
      flexion, or rotation 105, *246*, **739-**
  congenital 106, *252*, **758-**
Degeneration, degenerative
cerebellum 57, *91*, **355-**
cervical spine 102, *235*, **723-**
intervertebral disc (IV disk) 105, *246*, **739-**
lumbar (lumbosacral) 103, *239*, **7244**
thoracic spine 103, *239*, **7244**
Dehydration 44, *57*, **279-**
Delayed speech 109, *257*, **7845**
psychogenic 55, *86*, **316-**
Delay in development (physiological) 113, *294*, **7834**
mental 52, *74*, **315-**
Delinquency 53, *78*, **312-**
Delirium tremens 54, *80*, **3031**
Delivery (obstetrical)
with
  complication, any 94, *204*, **661-**
  fetopelvic disproportion 94, *204*, **661-**
  malpresentation 94, *204*, **661-**
  postpartum hemorrhage 94, *204*, **661-**
    delayed 94, *204*, **661-**
  premature delivery 93, *202*, **648-**
  outside of hospital 130, *371*, **V999**
    baby 107, *253*, **778-**
without complication normal 93, *203*, **650-**
Delusions 49, *67*, **295-**
Dementia NOS 49, *69*, **298-**
senile (presenile) 48, *66*, **294-**
Dendritic ulcer 33, *11*, **054-**
Dengue 37, *31*, **136-**
Dental
abnormalities 76, *148*, **520-**

caries or cysts 76, *148*, **520-**
Dependent on drugs 54, *83*, **3048**
Depression NOS 52, *72*, **3004**
anxiety 52, *72*, **3004**
endogenous 49, 68, **296-**
manic 49, *68*, **296-**
neurotic 52, *72*, **3004**
psychotic 49, *68*, **296-**
reactive 52, *72*, **3004**
  psychotic 49, *68*, **296-**
senile 48, *66*, **294-**
De Quervain's disease 102, *233*, **7263**
Derangement, knee 104, *244*, **717-**
acute, current injury 118, *312*, **836-**
chronic 104, *244*, **717-**
recurrent 105, *246*, **739-**
Dermatitis NOS 97, *214*, **692-**
actinic (sunburn) 97, *214*, **692-**
allergic 97, *214*, **692-**
atopic 96, *213*, **6918**
contact 97, *214*, **692-**
diaper 97, *215*, **6910**
due to
  adhesive plaster or tape 97, *214*, **692-**
  caterpillar 97, *214*, **692-**
  cosmetic 97, *214*, **692-**
  drug applied to skin 97, *214*, **692-**
  poison ivy 97, *214*, **692-**
  sunlight 97, *214*, **692-**
  weather, cold or hot 97, *214*, **692-**
exfoliative (neonatorum) 99, *227*, **709-**
factitial 98, *218*, **698-**
flexural 96, *213*, **6918**
herpetiformis 99, *227*, **709-**
hypostatic, lower extremities 68, *129*, **454-**
infectious eczematoid 96, *212*, **690-**
medicamentosa, applied to skin 97, *214*, **692-**
nummular 97, *214*, **692-**
pruritic 97, *214*, **692-**
purulent 95, *211*, **685-**
radiation (radium) (roentgen) (X-ray) 97, *214*, **692-**
Rhus 97, *214*, **692-**
seborrhoeic 96, *212*, **690-**
septic 95, *211*, **685-**
stasis 68, *129*, **454-**
suppurative 95, *211*, **685-**
vegetans 95, *211*, **685-**
Dermatofibroma 40, *41*, **216-**
Dermatographia 99, *226*, **708-**
Dermatomycosis 36, *24*, **110-**
Dermatomyositis 101, *231*, **725-**
Dermatophytosis 36, *24*, **110-**
Dermatosis
erythematosquamous 96, *212*, **690-**
papulos nigra 99, *227*, **709-**
precancerous 99, *227*, **709-**
progressive pigmentary 99, *227*, **709-**

Duodentis (cont.)
infective 77, 153, 536-
Dwarfism 44, 57, 279-
Dysentery
bacillary 31, 1, 008-
carrier 123, 339, V01-
NOS 31, 3, 009-
    presumed 31, 2, 009-
    proven 31, 1, 008-
Dysesthesia 109, 259, 7820
Dysfunction
brain 57, 91, 355-
hepatic 80, 165, 571-
ventricular 64, 188, 429-
Dysgraphia 115, 300, 7889
Dyshidrosis 98, 223, 705-
Dyskeratosis 99, 227, 709-
Dyslexia 52, 74, 315-
Dysmenorrhea 89, 191, 6253
Dysostosis cleidocranial 106, 252, 758-
Dyspareunia NOS 89, (374), 6250
male 86, 180, 607-
psychogenic 53, 79, 3027
Dyspepsia 77, 153, 536-
Dysphagia 115, 300, 7889
Dysplasia
acetabular 106, 248, 754-
cervical 87, 184, 622-
hip, congenital 106, 252, 758-
mammary, benign 86, 181, 610-
Dyspnea 111, 269, 7860
Dysuria 112, 286, 7881

Earache 60, 107, 388-
Ecchymosis NOS 69, 132, 459-
conjunctiva, spontaneous 58, 99, 378-
eye (eyelid), traumatic 121, 327, 929-
Eclampsia arising during pregnancy
        childbirth or puerperium 92, 199,
        642-
Ecthyma 95, 211, 685-
Ectopic
heartbeat ('nodal') 63, 115, 4276
pregnancy 91, 196, 633-
Ectropion
cervix 87, 184, 622-
eyelid 58, 99, 378-
Eczema NOS 97, 214, 692-
atopic 96, 213, 6918
external auditory meatus 59, 100, 3801
infantile 96, 213, 6918
marginatum 37, 31, 136-
seborrhoeic 96, 212, 690-
infantile 96, 213, 6918
vaccination (vaccinatum) 122, 336, 998-
Edema NOS 110, 265, 7823
allergic 122, (378), 9950
angioneurotic 122, (378), 9950
due to antifertility pill 122, (377), 9952

essential, acute 122, (378), 9950
hands 110, 265, 7823
legs NOS 110, 265, 7823
    due to obstruction 69, 132, 459-
pulmonary 75, 147, 519-
Edentulous 76, 148, 520-
Effects, adverse, of
chemicals, chiefly nonmedicinal 122, 335,
        989-
complications of
    medical care 122, 336, 998-
    surgery 122, 336, 998-
medicinal agents 122, (377), 9952
    overdose or wrong substance 122, 334,
        977-
physical agents (cold) (drowning)
        (heat) (lightning) 122, 337, 994-
sunlight 97, 214, 692-
Effort syndrome 51, 71, 3001
Effusion of
joint (chronic) 101, (289), 7190
pleura NOS 73, (5), 5119
    serofibrinous 73, (5), 5119
    tuberculous 31, 4, 011-
Elephantiasis 69, 132, 459-
filiarial 37, 28, 127-
Elevated
blood
    chemistry finding NEC 114, (51), 7902
    pressure without
        diagnosis of hypertension 115, (119),
        7962
hematologic finding NEC 114, 375, 7900
sedimentation rate 114, (375), 7900
urine test finding NEC 114, 298, 791-
Embolic CNS episode 57, 91, 355-
Embolism 67, 126, 443-
artery 67, 126, 443-
cerebral 66, 124, 438-
kidney 84, 174, 598-
multiple 67, 126, 443-
paradoxical 67, 126, 443-
pulmonary 67, 127, 415-
Emesis 111, 274, 787-
complicating pregnancy 93, 202, 648-
Emotional
instability 54, 84, 301-
upset 52, 73, 3009
Emphysema, pulmonary 74, 143, 492-
Empty sella syndrome 44, 57, 279-
Empyema 75, 147, 519-
Encephalitis NOS 57, 91, 355-
epidemic (sleeping sickness) 37, 31, 136-
equine 37, 31, 136-
herpes (simplex virus) 33, 11, 054-
lead 122, 335, 989-
Murray Valley (Australian) 37, 31, 136-
postinfective 37, 31, 136-
St. Louis 37, 31, 136-

Examination (*cont.*)
medical, with no disease detected 123, *338*, V70-
newborn (well baby) 123, *338*, V70-
postpartum 126, *352*, V24-
prenatal 126, *351*, V220
pre-operative 123, *338*, V70-
to rule out or exclude specific disease 123, *338*, V70-
X-ray 123, *338*, V70-
Exanthem, viral NEC 33, *14*, 057-
Exanthema subitum 33, *14*, 057-
Excessive sweating 113, *290*, 7808
Excoriation
due to injury 121, *326*, 918-
neurotic 98, *218*, 698
Exhaustion 113, *295*, 7807
Exophthalmos NOS 58, *99*, 378-
thyroid 42, *48*, 242-
Exostosis 102, *233*, 7263
Exotropia 58, *99*, 378-
Exposure (to)
chemical(s) 122, *335*, 989-
disease 123, *339*, V01-
Extrasystoles 63, *115*, 4276
Eye problems 58, *99*, 378-

Failure
heart, right or left sided 63, *112*, 428-
renal 84, *174*, 598-
respiratory 115, *300*, 7889
to thrive, in prenatal period 113, *294*, 7834
ventricular, left 63, *112*, 428-
Faint 110, *264*, 7802
Family history of disease 124, *342*, V10-
Family planning—*see* 124, *345*, V251
to 127, *347*, V256
Farmer's
lung 75, *147*, 519-
skin 97, *214*, 692-
Farsightedness 58, *94*, 367-
Fasciculation 109, *255*, 7810
Fasciitis, nodular 102, *234*, 728-
Fatigue 113, *295*, 7807
Favism 46, *60*, 282-
Fear 52, *73*, 3009
Fecal impaction 81, *167*, 579-
Feeding problem in baby 113, (*53*), 7833
Felon 95, *207*, 680-
Fertility, reduced 90, *195*, 606-
Fever
cat-scratch 37, *31*, 136-
glandular 34, *17*, 075-
from immunization 122, *336*, 998-
mosquito-borne 37, *31*, 136-
relapsing 37, *31*, 136-
rheumatic, acute 61, *108*, 390-
scarlet 32, *7*, 034-
unknown origin (FUO) 113, *291*, 7806

Fibrillation
atrial (auricular) 63, *113*, 4273
ventricular 64, *118*, 429-
Fibro-adenosis, breast 86, *181*, 610-
Fibrocystic breast 86, *181*, 610-
Fibroid uterus 40, *43*, 218-
Fibroma
prostate 85, *175*, 600-
skin 40, *41*, 216-
uterus 40, *43*, 216-
Fibroplasia, retrolental 58, *99*, 378-
Fibrosarcoma 39, *39*, 199-
Fibrosis
cystic 44, *57*, 279-
pulmonary 75, *147*, 519-
Fibrositis
shoulder 101, *232*, 7260
site, other NEC 102, *234*, 728–
Fifth disease 33, *14*, 057-
Fill out forms 125, *348*, V680
Fissure
anal 79, *162*, 565-
nipple 86, *182*, 611-
Fistula
anorectal 79, *162*, 565-
cutaneous 95, *211*, 685-
female genital tract 89, *194*, 629-
pilonidal 95, *211*, 685-
postoperative, persistent 122, *336*, 998-
rectovaginal 89, *194*, 629-
urethrovaginal 89, *194*, 629-
Fixation, joint 105, *246*, 739-
Flatfoot 104, *245*, 736-
Flatulence 112, *278*, 7873
Flexion contracture NEC 105, *246*, 739-
Floater 58, *99*, 378-
Floating
ribs 106, *252*, 758-
testes 86, *180*, 607-
Floppy larynx 75, *147*, 519-
Flu 72, *139*, 487-
Fluor (vaginalis) 89, *194*, 629-
Flushing 115, *300*, 7889
Flutter
atrial (auricular) 63, *113*, 4273
ventricular 64, *118*, 429-
Foley change 130, *371*, V999
Folliculitis 98, *222*, 704-
Food poisoning
Salmonella 31, *1*, 008-
specified bacteria 31, *1*, 008-
Staphylococcus 31, *1*, 008-
Foot drop 104, *245*, 736-
Forbes–Albright syndrome 44, *57*, 279-
Foreign body (in)
entering through orifice
anus 121, *331*, 939-
bronchus 121, *331*, 939-
ear 121, *331*, 939-

Infection (*cont.*)
umbilical 95, *211*, **685-**
  newborn 107, *253*, **778-**
urinary tract NOS 83, *170*, **595-**
  arising during pregnancy or
  puerperium 91, *198*, **6466**
vaginal 87, *185*, **6161**
viral, unspecified 35, *20*, **0799**
wound 121, *333*, **959-**
Infertility
female 90, *195*, **606-**
male 90, *195*, **606-**
Infestation
filarial 37, *28*, **127-**
helminths 37, *28*, **127-**
larvae 37, *29*, **132-**
leeches 37, *29*, **132-**
maggots 37, *29*, **132-**
mites 37, *30*, **133-**
pinworms 37, *28*, **127-**
ringworm 36, *24*, **110-**
sand fleas 37, *29*, **138-**
Strongyloides stercoratis 37, *28*, **127-**
tinea 36, *24*, **110-**
Infiltrate
chest or lung 75, *147*, **519-**
Inflamed, inflammation
lung 73, *140*, **486-**
skin 95, *211*, **685-**
Influenza 72, *139*, **487-**
gastric 31, *2*, **009-**
Influenza-like illness 72, *139*, **487-**
Ingested
foreign
  body 121, *330*, **930-**
  substance 122, *335*, **989-**
Ingrown
hair 98, *222*, **704-**
toenail 98, *221*, **703-**
Inhalation environmental risk 122, *335*,
  989-
Injury
blast, with internal injury 121, *333*, **959-**
crushing 121, *327*, **929-**
  internal injury 121, *333*, **959-**
eardrum 121, *333*, **959-**
  perforation 120, *323*, **889-**
internal 121, *333*, **959-**
  abdomen, chest, or pelvis 121, *333*, **959-**
intracranial 120, *322*, **850-**
  with skull fracture 116, *301*, **802-**
multiple 121, *333*, **959-**
teeth 120, *323*, **889-**
wound, open (laceration) 120, *323*, **889-**
Inoculation, prophylactic 123, *340*, **V03-**
Insomnia nonorganic origin 52, *75*,
  3074
Instability
ankle 105, *246*, **739-**
personality 54, *84*, **301-**

Instruction, health 126, *354*, **V654-**
education program 126, *354*, **V654-**
Insufficiency, insufficient
cardiac 63, *112*, **428-**
cerebrovascular 66, *124*, **438-**
coronary 62, *109*, **410-**
dietary 43, *52*, **260-**
food (nourishment) 122, *337*, **994-**
  due to economic problem—
    add code 127, *356*, **V602**
mental 55, *85*, **317-**
myocardial 63, *112*, **428-**
  with
    hypertension—*see* Hypertension
    rheumatic fever 61, *108*, **390-**
pancreatic 81, *167*, **579-**
pulmonary 75, *147*, **519-**
respiratory 111, *269*, **7860**
  in newborn 107, *253*, **778-**
valve, aortic or mitral 64, (*111*), **424-**
  rheumatic 61, *108*, **390-**
vascular 69, *132*, **459-**
venous 68, *129*, **454**
Intertrigo 99, *227*, **709-**
Intervertebral disc (disk) (degenerative)
  (prolapsed) (ruptured)
cervical 102, *235*, **723-**
lumbar (lumbosacral) 103, *239*, **7244**
thoracic 103, *239*, **7244**
Intestinal disease
infectious
  presumed 31, *2*, **009-**
  proven 31, *1*, **008-**
In-toeing 104, *245*, **736-**
Intolerance
food 81, *167*, **579-**
lactose 44, *57*, **279-**
Intoxication, alcohol
acute 54, *81*, **3050**
chronic 54, *80*, **3031**
Intussusception 81, *167*, **579-**
Inversion
foot 104, *245*, **736-**
nipple 86, *182*, **611-**
  puerperal 94, *205*, **676-**
Involuntary movements, abnormal 109,
  255, **7810**
Iritis 58, *99*, **378-**
Irregular
bowels 81, *167*, **579-**
menses 89, *190*, **6262**
pulse 64, *118*, **429-**
Irritable colon or bowel syndrome 78, *159*,
  558-
Irritation
bladder 84, *174*, **598-**
cervical 87, *184*, **622-**
eye 58, *99*, **378-**
nervous 115, *300*, **7889**

Irritation (*cont.*)
nose 75, *147*, **519-**
rectal 81, *167*, **579-**
vagina 89, *194*, **629-**
Ischemia, ischemic
attack, transient 66, *123*, **435-**
heart disease
  asymptomatic 62, *110*, **412-**
  chronic 62, *110*, **412-**
  subacute 62, *109*, **410-**
leg, Volkmann's (with peroneal nerve
  injury) 121, *333*, **959-**
peripheral vascular condition 67, *126*, **443-**
  due to ergot ingestion-code also 122,
  334, **977-**
Itch
barbers' 36, *24*, **110-**
eye(s) 58, *99*, **378-**
filarial 37, *28*, **127-**
grain 37, *30*, **133-**
groin 36, *24*, **110-**
grocers' 37, *30*, **133-**
harvest 37, *30*, **133-**
NOS 98, *218*, **698-**
rectal 98, *218*, **698-**
seven-year 128, *359*, **V611**
  meaning acariasis, scabies or chiggers
  37, *30*, **133-**
swimmers' 37, *88*, **127-**
vaginal 98, *218*, **698-**
washerwomen's 97, *214*, **692-**
water 37, *28*, **127-**
winter 98, *218*, **698-**

Jacksonian seizure (epilepsy) 56, *89*, **345-**
Jaundice NOS 115, *300*, **7889**
acholuric 46, *60*, **282-**
epidemic 34, *15*, **070-**
  leptospiral or spirochetal 37, *31*, **136-**
hemolytic 46, *61*, **285-**
infectious 34, *15*, **070-**
from injection, inoculation, or
  transfusion 34, *15*, **070-**
obstructive 81, *166*, **574-**
Jealousy 53, *78*, **312-**
Jerks, myoclonic 57, *91*, **355-**

Keloid 99, *227*, **709-**
Keratitis 58, *99*, **378-**
Keratoderma 99, *227*, **709-**
Keratosis
actinic 99, *227*, **709-**
blennorrhagica 99, *227*, **709-**
follicular (nevus) 106, *252*, **758-**
punctata 99, *227*, **709-**
seborrhoeic 99, *227*, **709-**
senilis (solar) 99, *227*, **709-**
solar 99, *227*, **709-**

Kidney stone 83, *171*, **592-**
Kimmelstiel–Wilson syndrome 43, *50*, **250-**
  and 82, *168*, **580-**
Kleptomania 53, *78*, **312-**
Klinefelter's syndrome 106, *252*, **758-**
Klippel–Feil syndrome (brevicollis) 106,
  252, **758-**
Knock knee 104, *245*, **736-**
Knots, surfer (knee) (knobs) 121, *326*, **918-**
Koilonychia 98, *221*, **703-**
Korsakoff's psychosis (nonalcoholic) 48,
  66, **294-**
alcoholic 54, *80*, **3031**
Kraurosis
ani 81, *167*, **579-**
penis 86, *186*, **607-**
vagina or vulva 89, *194*, **629-**
Kummell's disease or spondylitis 102, *237*,
  721-
Kussmaul's
coma 43, *50*, **250-**
disease 69, *132*, **459-**
Kyphosis, kyphoscoliosis
acquired 103, *240*, **737-**
adolescent (postural) 103, *240*, **737-**
adult 103, *240*, **737-**
congenital 106, *252*, **758-**
late effect of polio 32, *8*, **045-** and 103, *240*,
  737-
pelvis 105, *246*, **739-**
senile 103, *240*, **737-**
tuberculous 31, *4*, **011-**

Labor
false 93, *202*, **648-**
missed 94, *204*, **661-**
premature 93, *202*, **648-**
with complications 94, *204*, **661-**
  dead fetus under 28 weeks' gestation
  93, *201*, **634-**
Labyrinthitis acute (circumscribed)
  (destructive) (purulent) 60, *104*,
  386-
Laceration
cerebral 120, *322*, **850-**
cervix, old 87, *184*, **622-**
delivery complication 94, *204*, **661-**
head 120, *323*, **889-**
infected 121, *333*, **959-**
internal organs of abdomen, chest, or
  pelvis, due to injury 121, *333*, **959-**
late effect of 121, *332*, **908-**
limb(s), upper or lower 120, *323*, **889-**
multiple locations 120, *323*, **889-**
neck 120, *323*, **889-**
nerve 121, *333*, **959-**
trunk 120, *323*, **889-**
with foreign body in tissue 120, *323*, **889-**
  superficial injury 121, *329*, **912-**

Neoplasm, benign (*cont.*)
  breast 40, *42*, **217-**
  gastrointestinal tract 41, *45*, **229-**
  hemangioma 41, *44*, **228-**
  lipoma 40, *40*, **214-**
  lymphangioma 41, *44*, **228-**
  site, other NEC 41, *45*, **229-**
  skin 40, *41*, **216-**
  uterus (cervix uteri) 40, *43*, **218-**
  in situ 39, *39*, **199-**
    cervix 39, *36*, **180-**
  malignant
    adnexa 39, *39*, **199-**
    anus 38, *32*, **151-**
    basal cell 38, *34*, **173-**
    bladder 39, *37*, **188-**
    breast 38, *35*, **174-**
    bronchus 38, *33*, **162-**
    cervix 39, *36*, **180-**
    colon 38, *32*, **151-**
    endometrium 39, *36*, **180-**
    epiglottis 38, *33*, **162-**
    esophagus 38, *32*, **151-**
    face 39, *39*, **199-**
      squamous cell 38, *34*, **173-**
    gastrointestinal tract 38, *32*, **151-**
    genital tract
      female 39, *36*, **180-**
      male 39, *37*, **188-**
    Hodgkin's 39, *38*, **201-**
    kidney 39, *37*, **188-**
    larynx 38, *33*, **162-**
    leukemia 39, *38*, **201-**
    lung 38, *33*, **162-**
    lymphoma 39, *38*, **201-**
    melanoma 38, *34*, **173-**
    multiple myeloma 39, *38*, **201-**
    ovary 39, *36*, **180-**
    pancreas 39, *39*, **199-**
    prostate 39, *37*, **188-**
    skin 38, *34*, **173-**
    stomach 38, *32*, **151-**
    subcutaneous tissue 38, *34*, **173-**
    testis 39, *37*, **188-**
    uterus 39, *36*, **180-**
    vagina 39, *36*, **180-**
    vulva 39, *36*, **180-**
Nephritis
arising during pregnancy 93, *202*, **648-**
chronic 84, *174*, **598-**
glomerulonephritis 82, *168*, **580-**
interstitial, diffuse 82, *168*, **580-**
lupus 101, *231*, **725-**
pyelonephritis 82, *169*, **5901**
salt-losing 84, *174*, **598-**
Nephrocalcinosis 44, *57*, **279-**
Nephrolithiasis 83, *171*, **592-**
Nephropathy 82, *168*, **580-**
sickle cell 46, *60*, **282-**

Nephrosclerosis 65, *121*, **402-**
due to hypertension 65, *121*, **402-**
gouty 44, *54*, **274-**
malignant 65, *121*, **402-**
Nephrotic syndrome 82, *168*, **580-**
arising during pregnancy 98, *202*, **648-**
Nervousness 115, *300*, **7889**
Nervous stomach 51, *71*, **3001**
Neuralgia 57, *91*, **355-**
occipital 57, *91*, **355-**
trigeminal 57, *91*, **355-**
Neurasthenia 52, *73*, **3009**
cardiac 51, *71*, **3001**
Neuritis 102, *234*, **728-**
Neurocirculatory asthenia 51, *71,* **3001**
Neurodermatitis 98, *218*, **698-**
atopic 96, *213*, **6918**
diffuse 96, *213*, **6918**
disseminated 96, *213*, **6918**
psychogenic 51, *71*, **3001**
Neurofibroma 41, *45*, **229-**
Neurofibromatosis 41, *46*, **239-**
malignant 39, *39*, **199-**
Neuroma 41, *45*, **229-**
digital 57, *91*, **355-**
intermetatarsal 57, *91*, **355-**
Morton's 57, *91*, **355-**
Neuromuscular disease 57, *91*, **355-**
Neuromyasthenia (epidemic) 37, *31*, **136-**
Neuronitis, vestibular 60, *104*, **386-**
Neuropathy 57, *91*, **355-**
alcoholic 54, *80*, **3031**
diabetic 43, *50*, **250-** and 57, *91*, **355-**
peripheral 57, *91*, **355-**
sciatic 57, *91*, **355-**
  associated with diabetes 43, *50*, **250-** and
    57, *91*, **355-**
ulnar 57, *91*, **355-**
Neurosis
anxiety 50, *70*, **3000**
cardiac 51, *71*, **3001**
combat 53, *77*, **308-**
depersonalization 52, *73*, **3009**
depressive (reaction) 52, *72*, **3004**
hypochondriacal 51, *71*, **3001**
hysterical
  conversion 51, *71*, **3001**
  dissociative 51, *71*, **3001**
neurasthenic 52, *73*, **3009**
obsessive–compulsive 52, *73*, **3009**
occupational 52, *73*, **3009**
phobic 52, *73*, **3009**
respiratory 51, *71*, **3001**
unspecified 52, *73*, **3009**
Neurosyphilis 35, *22*, **090-**
Neutropenia 46, *64*, **288-**
Nevus NEC 40, *41*, **216-**
acneiformis unilateralis 106, *252*, **758-**
amelanotic (nonpigmented) 40, *41*, **216-**

Osteomyelitis NOC (*cont.*)
focal 105, *246*, **739-**
sclerosing 105, *246*, **739-**
suppurative 105, *246*, **739-**
Osteoporosis 104, *243*, **7330**
postmenopausal 104, *243*, **7330**
post-traumatic 105, *246*, **739-**
senile 104, *243*, **7330**
Osteosarcoma 39, *39*, **199-**
Otalgia 60, *107*, **388-**
Otitis NOS 59, *101*, **3820**
acute
    secretory (nonsuppurative) 59, *102*, **3811**
    suppurative 59, *101*, **3820**
chronic 59, *101*, **3820**
externa 59, *100*, **3801**
    tropical 36, *24*, **110-**
exudative, chronic 59, *102*, **3811**
nonsuppurative 59, *102*, **3811**
serous, chronic 59, *102*, **3811**
suppurative 59, *101*, **3820**
    chronic 60, *107*, **388-**
unspecified 59, *101*, **3820**
with mastoiditis—code both
Otopathy 60, *107*, **388-**
Otorrhea 60, *107*, **388-**
Otosclerosis 60, *105*, **382-**
Otto's disease of pelvis 100, *229*, **715-**
Overactive thyroid 42, *48*, **242-**
Overbite 76, *148*, **520-**
Overdevelopment, breast 86, *182*, **611-**
Overeating 115, *300*, **7889**
nonorganic origin 55, *86*, **316-**
Overexertion 122, *337*, **994-**
Overexposure 122, *337*, **994-**
Overlapping toe 104, *245*, **736-**
Overweight 44, *55*, **278-**
Overwork 113, *295*, **7807**
Ovulation (cycle)
failure or lack of 90, *195*, **606-**
pain 89, *191*, **6253**
Oxyuriasis 37, *28*, **127-**
Ozena 75, *147*, **519-**

Pacemaker
functioning prosthesis 124, *342*, **V10-**
    patient care management 124, *342*, **V10-**
malfunctioning prosthesis 122, *336*, **998-**
wandering 64, *118*, **429-**
Pachyderma 99, *227*, **709-**
Paget's disease 105, *246*, **739-**
breast (extramammary) 38, *35*, **174-**
malignant 38, *35*, **174-**
osteitis deformans 105, *246*, **739-**
scrotum 38, *34*, **173-**
skin 38, *34*, **173-**
Pain(s)
abdominal 112, *279*, **7890**
adnexal 89, *193*, **6269**

anus 79, *163*, **5646**
arch 102, (*286*), **7295**
arm 102, (*286*), **7295**
axillary 112, *278*, **7873**
back 103, *238*, **7242**
    postsurgical 103, *238*, **7242**
    psychogenic 53, *76*, **3078**
    with radiating symptoms 103, *239*, **7244**
bladder 115, *300*, **7889**
breast 86, *182*, **611-**
chest 110, *262*, **7865**
coccyx 103, *238*, **7242**
ear 60, *107*, **388-**
epigastrium 112, *279*, **7890**
extremity 102, (*286*), **7295**
eye 58, *99*, **378-**
facial 109, *258*, **7840**
    atypical 57, *91*, **355-**
finger 102, (*286*), **7295**
flank 112, *279*, **7890**
foot 102, (*286*), **7295**
gas (intestinal) 112, *278*, **7873**
genital organs
    female 89, *194*, **629-**
    male 86, *180*, **607-**
generalized 115, *300*, **7889**
groin 112, *279*, **7890**
'growing' 112, *279*, **7890**
head 109, *258*, **7840**
hip 101, (*288*), **7194**
intermenstrual 89, *191*, **6253**
jaw 76, *148*, **520-**
joint 101, (*288*), **7194**
leg or limb 102, (*286*), **7295**
lumbar region 103, *238*, **7242**
micturition 115, *300*, **7889**
muscle 102, *234*, **728-**
nasopharynx 75, *147*, **519-**
neck 102, *235*, **723-**
    of mental origin 53, *76*, **3078**
ovulation 89, *191*, **6253**
penis 86, *180*, **607-**
periarticular 101, (*288*), **7194**
pleuritic 110, *262*, **7865**
precordial 110, *262*, **7865**
psychogenic origin, in any site or body
    system 53, *76*, **3078**
radicular 102, *234*, **728-**
rectal 79, *163*, **5646**
rib 115, *300*, **7889**
sacroiliac 103, *238*, **7242**
scapula 102, (*286*), **7295**
shoulder 102, (*286*), **7295**
stomach 77, *153*, **536-**
temporomandibular 109, *258*, **7840**
thoracic 103, *238*, **7242**
toe 102, (*286*), **7295**
urinary system 115, *300*, **7889**
vertebrogenic (syndrome) 103, *238*, **7242**

Pregnancy (*cont.*)
with
  complicated delivery 94, *204*, **661-**
  eclampsia or pre-eclampsia 92, *199*, **642-**
  toxemia 92, *199*, **642-**
  uncomplicated delivery 93, *203*, **650-**
  urinary infection 91, *198*, **6466**
Pre-infarction syndrome 62, *109*, **410-**
Premature, prematurity
beat
  atrial 63, *115*, **4276**
  A-V nodal (junctional) 63, *115*, **4276**
  nodal 63, *115*, **4276**
  ventricular 63, *115*, **4276**
contractions, heart 63, *115*, **4276**
delivery—*see* Delivery
ejaculation 51, *71*, **3001**
heartbeats 63, *115*, **4276**
menopause 44, *57*, **279-**
newborn 107, *253*, **778-**
puberty 44, *57*, **279-**
senility 44, *57*, **279-**
systoles 63, *115*, **4276**
Premenstrual tension syndrome 88, *188*,
  6254
Prenatal care 126, *351*, **V220**
Presbyacusis 60, *107*, **388-**
Presbyopia 58, *94*, **367-**
Prescription
given without need for examination or
  interview 125, *348*, **V680**
oral contraceptive 124, *344*, **V255**
Presenility NOS 44, *57*, **279-**
dementia 48, *66*, **294-**
Pressure
intraocular 58, *99*, **378-**
sore 99, *225*, **707-**
Priapism 86, *180*, **607-**
Prickly
heat 88, *223*, **705-**
sensation 109, *259*, **7820**
Primipara, old, complicating delivery 94,
  204, **661-**
Problems(s), individual and family
aged parents or in-laws 128, *361*, **V613**
alcohol abuse 54, *80*, **3031**
attitudes or behavior that prevent adequate
  therapy 130, *369*, **V629**
caring for family member 128, *358*, **V614**
  offspring 128, *360*, **V612**
  parent 128, *360*, **V612**
  spouse 128, *359*, **V611**
cosmetic NEC 130, *371*, **V999**
customs or beliefs that interfere with
  therapy 130, *369*, **V629**
deprivation
  cultural 129, *366*, **V624**
  economic 127, *356*, **V602**
  education 129, *364*, **V623**

discrimination
  physical
    appearance 129, *366*, **V624**
    disability for job opportunity 130, *367*,
      V620
  political 129, *366*, **V624**
  religious 129, *366*, **V624**
disruption in family life 129, *362*, **V610**
divorce 129, *362*, **V610**
drug or marihuana abuse
  parent–child relation 128, *360*, **V612**
  spouse 128, *359*, **V611**
economic 127, *356*, **V602**
education and school
  delinquency (severe) 53, *78*, **312-** and
    129, *364*, **V623**
  discouragement 129, *364*, **V623**
  dissatisfaction 129, *364*, **V623**
  dropout 129, *364*, **V623**
  need for job training 129, *364*, **V623**
  selection of career 130, *367*, **V620**
  work too difficult 129, *364*, **V623**
family
  disruption 129, *362*, **V610**
  relationship NEC 129, *363*, **V619**
financial 127, *356*, **V602**
  as it affects legal proceedings 130, (*370*),
    V625
housing 127, *357*, **V600**
  eviction notice 127, *357*, **V600**
  forced out by urban renewal 127, *357*,
    V600
  inadequate facilities 127, *357*, **V600**
  lack of heat 127, *357*, **V600**
intervention by relatives in family
  relationship 129, *363*, **V619**
isolation, social 129, *366*, **V624**
language barrier
  occupational 130, *367*, **V620**
  social—*see* 129, *366*, **V624** and 130, *369*,
    V629
legal 130, (*370*), **V625**
  divorce 129, *362*, **V610**
  imprisonment 130, (*370*), **V625**
  insurance settlement 130, (*370*), **V625**
  juvenile delinquency (court)—*see* 53, *78*,
    312- and 129, *364*, **V623** or 130,
    (*370*), **V625**
  legal investigations 130, (*370*), **V625**
  litigation 130, (*370*), **V625**
    divorce 129, *362*, **V610**
  nonpayment of child support 127, *356*,
    V602
  separation 129, *362*, **V610**
living alone
  loneliness 129, *366*, **V624**
    grief reaction 53, *77*, **308-**
  need for housekeeper or nursing aide
    130, *369*, **V629**

Rupture, ruptured (*cont.*)
venous 68, *129*, **454-**

Salmonella 31, *1*, **008-**
carrier 123, *339*, **V01-**
Salpingitis
acute or chronic 87, *183*, **614-**
ear 59, *103*, **3815**
eustachian 59, *103*, **3815**
gonococcal 36, *23*, **098-**
Salpingo-oophoritis—*see* Salpingitis
Salt-losing syndrome 84, *174*, **598-**
Sarcoidosis 37, *31*, **136-**
Scabies 37, *30*, **133-**
Scalds 121, *328*, **949-**
Scalenus anticus syndrome 57, *91*, **355-**
Scar formation following injury 121, *332*, **908-**
Scarlatina 32, *7*, **034-**
Scarlet fever 32, *7*, **034-**
Scheuermann's disease 104, *242*, **732-**
Schistosomiasis 37, *28*, **127-**
Schizophrenia, all types 49, *67*, **295-**
Schmorl's nodes 105, *246*, **739-**
School phobia in child 129, *364*, **V623**
Sciatica
associated with diabetes 43, *50*, **250-** and 57, *91*, **355-**
possible intervertebral disc 103, *239*, **7244**
traumatic 103, *239*, **7244**
Scleroderma 101, *231*, **725-**
Sclerosis
arteriosclerosis, heart 62, *110*, **412-**
cardiovascular 62, *110*, **412-**
endocardial 62, *110*, **412-**
multiple 56, *87*, **340-**
renal 84, *174*, **598-**
Scoliosis
congenital 106, *252*, **758-**
idiopathic 103, *240*, **737-**
nonstructual 103, *240*, **737-**
paralytic 103, *240*, **737-**
postural 103, *240*, **737-**
Scotoma 58, *99*, **378-**
Scratch, skin 121, *326*, **918-**
Scurvy 43, *52*, **260-**
Sebaceous
cyst 98, *220*, **7062**
wen 98, *220*, **7062**
Seborrhoea 99, *227*, **709-**
Seizure NOS 109, *254*, **7803-**
epileptic (akinetic) (myoclonic) 56, *89*, **345-**
febrile 109, *254*, **7803**
grand mal 56, *89*, **345-**
hysterical 51, *71*, **3001**
Jacksonian 56, *89*, **345-**
petit mal 56, *89*, **345-**
Senescence 114, *297*, **797-**

Senility without psychosis 114, *297*, **797-**
Separation
epiphysis, traumatic—code as fracture joint
knee or patella 118, *312*, **836-**
site, other NEC 119, *313*, **839-**
Sepsis, umbilical cord 107, *253*, **778-**
Septicemia 37, *31*, **136-**
puerperal 94, *206*, **670-**
Serology
false positive 115, *299*, **793-**
positive 35, *22*, **090-**
Serum sickness 122, *336*, **998-**
Sexual
counseling 126, *354*, **V654-**
deviation 55, *86*, **316-**
problems NEC 130, *371*, **V999**—*see also* 53, *79*, **3027**
Shigellosis (dysentery) 31, *1*, **008-**
Shingles 32, *10*, **053-**
Shock
anaphylactic, due to
drugs (medications) 122, *334*, **977-**
serum or inoculation 122, *334*, **977-**
electric 122, *337*, **994-**
following injury 121, *333*, **959-**
insulin 44, *57*, **279-**
lightning 122, *337*, **994-**
Short
breath 111, *269*, **7860**
hamstring 105, *246*, **739-**
leg
acquired 104, *245*, **736-**
congenital 106, *248*, **754-**
sight 58, *94*, **367-**
Shoulder-hand syndrome 57, *91*, **355-**
Sickle cell anemia or trait 46, *60*, **282-**
Sickness
air travel 122, *337*, **994-**
altitude 122, *337*, **994-**
car 122, *337*, **994-**
motion 122, *337*, **994-**
sleeping 37, *31*, **136-**
travel 122, *337*, **994-**
Sever's disease 104, *242*, **732-**
Sinus
arrest 64, *118*, **429-**
arrhythmia 64, *118*, **429-**
pauses 64, *118*, **429-**
Sinusitis, acute or chronic 70, *134*, **461-**
Sixth disease 33, *14*, **057-**
Sjogren's syndrome 101, *231*, **725-**
Sleep
disorder, psychogenic 52, *75*, **3074**
walking 52, *75*, **3074**
Slipped disc (disk)
cervical 102, *235*, **723-**
lumbar (lumbosacral) 103, *238*, **7242**
thoracic 103, *238*, **7242**

State—*see* Neurosis
Status
arthrodesis 124, *342*, **V10-**
asthmaticus 74, *144*, **493-**
colostomy 124, *342*, **V10-**
epilepticus 56, *89*, **345-**
post-cataract 124, *342*, **V10-**
postmyocardial infarction 62, *110*, **412-**
post survey 124, *342*, **V10-**
Stave—*see also* Fracture
thumb 117, *307*, **814-**
Steatorrhea, idiopathic 81, *167*, **579-**
Stein–Leventhal syndrome 44, *57*, **279-**
Stenosis
aortic 64, *(111)*, **424-**
rheumatic 61, *108*, **390-**
cervical 87, *184*, **622-**
colostomy 81, *167*, **579-**
meatal 84, *174*, **598-**
mitral 61, *108*, **390-**
congenital 106, *247*, **746-**
nonrheumatic 64, *(111)*, **424-**
pulmonary 106, *247*, **746-**
pyloric 77, *153*, **536-**
congenital 106, *252*, **758-**
spinal 105, *246*, **739-**
tearduct 58, *99*, **378-**
congenital 106, *251*, **7436**
urethral 84, *174*, **598-**
vaginal 89, *194*, **629-**
Sterility, female or male 90, *195*, **606-**
Sterilization (female) (male)
advice on 125, *347*, **V256**
family planning procedure 124, *343*, **V252**
Stiff
joint NEC 101, *(288)*, **7194**
surgical fusion 124, *342*, **V10-**
neck—*see* torticollis 124, *342*, **V10-**
Still birth 107, *253*, **778-**
Sting—*see also* Bites
ant 120, *325*, **910-**
bee, hornet, or wasp 120, *325*, **910-**
fish 120, *325*, **910-**
plant 97, *214*, **692-**
venomous
animal 122, *335*, **989-**
insect 120, *325*, **910-**
Stomatitis
aphthous (canker sore) (ulcerative) 76, *149*, **528-**
epidemic 37, *31*, **136-**
herpes 33, *11*, **054-**
mycotic 36, *25*, **112-**
parasitic 36, *25*, **112-**
Vincent's 37, *31*, **136-**
Strabismus 58, *99*, **378-**
Straight-back cardiovascular syndrome 106, *252*, **758-**
Strain—*see also* Sprain

eye 58, *99*, **378-**
old
back 105, *246*, **739-**
lumbar (sacroiliac) joint 102, *234*, **728-**
Streptococcal sore throat 32, *7*, **034-**
Streptoderma 95, *211*, **685-**
Stress
chronic—*see* Problem(s)
incontinence 88, *186*, **618-**
male 112, *281*, **7883**
Stretch marks 99, *227*, **709-**
Stricture
cervix 88, *187*, **627-**
ureter 84, *174*, **598-**
urethra 84, *174*, **598-**
Stridor 111, *269*, **7860**
congenital 106, *252*, **758-**
laryngeal 106, *252*, **758-**
Striae atrophicae 99, *227*, **709-**
Stroke syndrome 66, *124*, **438-**
Stuttering (psychogenic) 55, *86*, **316-**
Sty (stye) (external) (internal) 57, *93*, **3730**
Subendocardial infarction 62, *109*, **410-**
Subluxation
hip, congenital 106, *248*, **754-**
traumatic
knee 118, *312*, **836-**
patella 118, *312*, **836-**
site, other NEC 119, *313*, **839-**
Suicide tendency 52, *73*, **3009**
Sunburn 97, *214*, **692-**
Sunstroke 122, *337*, **994-**
Supernumerary nipples 106, *252*, **758-**
Suppression, lactation 94, *205*, **676-**
Surfer knots (knees) (knobs) 121, *326*, **918-**
Surgical assists 126, *353*, **V50-**
Sweating, excessive 113, *290*, **7808**
Swelling
abdomen NOS 114, *296*, **7822**
allergy 122, *(378)*, **9950**
arm 102, *(286)*, **7295**
breast 86, *182*, **611-**
face 114, *296*, **7822**
foot 102, *(286)*, **7295**
gland 110, *266*, **7856**
joint 101, *(289)*, **7190**
leg 102, *(286)*, **7295**
localized 114, *296*, **7822**
not yet diagnosed 114, *296*, **7822**
pelvis 114, *296*, **7822**
penis 86, *180*, **607-**
scrotum 86, *180*, **607-**
Swimmer's ear 59, *100*, **3801**
Symblepharon 58, *99*, **378-**
Syncope NOS 110, *264*, **7802**
cardiac 110, *264*, **7802**
carotid sinus 57, *91*, **355-**
due to lumbar puncture (tap) 122, *336*, **998-**
tussive 111, *270*, **7862**

Torsion
testis 86, *180*, **607-**
tibial 104, *245*, **736-**
Torticollis
acquired 102, *235*, **723-**
   traumatic, current 120, *319*, **8470**
congenital 106, *252*, **758-**
spasmodic (wry neck) 57, *91*, **355-**
Toxemia
affecting fetus or newborn 107, *253*, **778-**
of pregnancy or puerperium 92, *199*, **642-**
Toxicity to
carbon monoxide 122, *335*, **989-**
food—*see* Poisoning
industrial materials 122, *335*, **989-**
medicinal agents (drugs) 122, *334*, **977-**
mushrooms, noxious 122, *335*, **989-**
nonmedical chemicals 122, *335*, **989-**
ozone 122, *335*, **989-**
poisonous plants 122, *335*, **989-**
Toxoplasmosis 37, *31*, **136-**
Tracheitis
acute 71, *137*, **464-**
chronic 74, *142*, **491-**
Tracheobronchitis 72, *138*, **466-**
Tracheopharyngitis 70, *133*, **460-**
Trachoma 37, *31*, **136-**
Transfusion 130, *371*, **V999**
Transient
cerebral ischemia 66, *123*, **435-**
ischemic attack 66, *123*, **435-**
Transplant requiring observation or care
   124, *342*, **V10-**
Transvestitism 55, *86*, **316-**
Trauma—*see* Injury
Trematode infestation 37, *28*, **127-**
Tremor NOS 109, *255*, **7810**
benign essential 57, *91*, **355-**
familial 57, *91*, **355-**
hysterical 51, *71*, **3001**
senilis 114, *297*, **797-**
Trench
fever 37, *31*, **136-**
foot 122, *337*, **994-**
mouth 37, *31*, **136-**
Trichiasis 98, *222*, **704-**
Trichiniasis, trichinosis 37, *28*, **127-**
Trichomonas, trichomoniasis, proven
   infection
urogenital 37, *27*, **1310**
vaginalis 37, *27*, **1310**
Trigger finger 102, *233*, **7263**
Trigonitis 83, *170*, **595-**
Truancy, childhood 53, *78*, **312-**
with education problem—code also 129,
   364, **V623**
Tubercule, Darwin's 106, *252*, **758-**
Tuberculosis
all sites 31, *4*, **011-**

contact with 123, *339*, **V01-**
late effects 31, *4*, **011-**
positive conversion test 31, *4*, **011-**
Tularemia 37, *31*, **136-**
Tussive syncope 111, *270*, **7862**
Tympanic membrane rupture
nontraumatic history 60, *107*, **388-**
traumatic 120, *323*, **889-**
Tympanitis 60, *107*, **388-**
Tympanosclerosis 60, *107*, **388-**
Typhoid 31, *1*, **008-**
carrier (state) 123, *339*, **V01-**
Typhus (endemic) (epidemic) 37, *31*, **136-**

Ulcer
aphthous, oral (stomatitis) 76, *199*, **528-**
cervix 87, *184*, **622-**
chronic, varicose, of leg 68, *129*, **454-**
corneal 58, *99*, **378-**
Curling's—*see* 76, *151*, **532-** and 76, *152*,
   533-
decubitus 99, *225*, **707-**
dendritic 33, *11*, **054-**
duodenal 76, *151*, **532-**
gastric 76, *152*, **533-**
gastrojejunal 76, *152*, **533-**
Hunner's 83, *170*, **595-**
hypertensive or ischemic, or legs 99, *225*,
   707- and code also the
   hypertension
lower extremity
   atrophic 99, *225*, **707-**
   chronic 99, *225*, **707-**
   decubitus 99, *225*, **707-**
   pyogenic 99, *225*, **707-**
   varicose 68, *129*, **454-**
marginal (anastomotic) (stomal) 76, *152*,
   533-
nose 75, *147*, **519-**
palate 76, *149*, **528-**
penis 86, *180*, **607-**
peptic 76, *152*, **533-**
pyloric 76, *152*, **533-**
rodent (skin) 38, *34*, **173-**
skin 99, *225*, **707-**
stasis, varicose 68, *129*, **454-**
stomal (gastrojejunal) 76, *152*, **533-**
trophic, decubitus 99, *225*, **707-**
tropical 99, *225*, **707-**
varicose 68, *129*, **454-**
with gangrene—code also 115, *300*, **7889**
Underdevelopment, physiologic 113, *294*,
   7834
Underweight NOS 113, *294*, **7834**
due to
   feeding problem in baby 113, (*53*), **7833**
   weight loss 113, *293*, **7832**
Undescended testicle 106, *249*, **7525**
Unmarried parenthood female 129, *365*, **V616**

Vomiting NOS 111. *274*, **7870**
allergic 77, *153*, **536-**
arising during pregnancy 93, *202*, **648-**
blood 79, (*276*), **578-**
causing asphyxia, choking, or
    suffocation 121, *331*, **939**
cyclical 77, *153*, **536-**
    psychogenic 51, *71*, **3001**
functional 77, *153*, **536-**
hysterical or nervous 51, *71*, **3001**
pernicious 77, *153*, **536-**
    of pregnancy 93, *202*, **648-**
physiological 111, *274*, **7870**
Von Gierke's disease 44, *57*, **279-**
Von Recklinghausen's disease 41, *46*, **239-**
bones 44, *57*, **279-**
Voyeurism 55, *86*, **316-**
Vulvitis (acute) (chronic) (senile) 87, *185*,
    6161
blenrorrhagic 36, *23*, **098-**
leukoplakic 87, *185*, **6161**
monilial 36, *26*, **1121**
syphilitic 35, *22*, **090-**
Vulvovaginitis 87, *185*, **6161**

Walking in sleep 52, *75*, **3074**
Wandering pacemaker 64, *118*, **429-**
Wart (common) (filiform) (infectious)
    (viral) 35, *19*, **0781**
plantar 35, *19*, **0781**
prosector 31, *4*, **011-**
seborrhoeic 99, *227*, **709-**
senile 99, *227*, **709-**
soft 99, *227*, **709-**
'venereal' 35, *19*, **0781**
water 37, *31*, **136-**
Water
deprivation 122, *337*, **994-**
intoxication 44, *57*, **279-**
Wax in ear 60, *106*, **3804**
Weak, weakness NOS 113, *295*, **7807**
joint 105, *246*, **739-**
limb 105, *246*, **739-**
muscle 102, *234*, **728-**
newborn 107, *253*, **778-**
senile 114, *297*, **797-**
Weather
effects of NEC 122, *337*, **994-**
skin 97, *214*, **692-**
Weight loss 113, *293*, **7832**
Well baby, care of examination 123, *338*,
    V70-
Wen 98, *220*, **7062**
Wheal 99, *227*, **709-**
Wheezing 111, *269*, **7860**
'Whiplash' injury (neck) 120, *319*, **8470**
Whisper speech 109, *257*, **7845**

Whooping cough 32, *6*, **033-**
Withdrawal syndrome (drug) (narcotic)
    54, *83*, **3048**
Wolf–Parkinson–White syndrome
paroxysmal tachycardia 63, *114*, **4270**
other 64, *118*, **429-**
Worms 37, *28*, **127-**
Wound
open (by firearms) (cutting) (ligament)
    (muscle) (penetrating) (perforating)
    (tendon)
    abdominal wall 120, *323*, **889-**
    animal bite 120, *323*, **889-**
    cerebral 120, *322*, **850-**
    eye 120, *323*, **889-**
    foot 120, *323*, **889-**
    groin or flank 120, *323*, **889-**
    infected 121, *333*, **959-**
    hand 120, *323*, **889-**
    head 120, *323*, **889-**
    infected 121, *333*, **959-**
    internal organ of abdomen, chest, or pelvis
        (heart) (intestine)
        (liver) (lungs) 121, *333*, **959-**
    limb (lower) (upper) 120, *323*, **889-**
    neck 120, *323*, **889-**
    trunk 120, *323*, **889-**
        internal organ 121, *333*, **959-**
    with foreign body in tissue 120, *323*, **889-**
        superficial 121, *329*, **912-**
    superficial 121, *326*, **918-**
        insect bite 120, *325*, **910-**
Wrinkling of facial skin 99, *227*, **709-**
Wrist drop 104, *245*, **736-**
Wry neck 102, *235*, **723-**
Wucheria infestation 37, *28*, **127-**

Xanthelasma 44, *56*, **272-**
Xeroderma 106, *252*, **758-**
Xerosis 99, *227*, **709-**
Xerostomia 76, *149*, **528-**
X-ray
abnormal findings, not yet diagnosed 115,
    299, **793-**
adverse effects of
    due to
        inadvertent exposure 122, *337*, **994-**
        therapy complication 122, *337*, **994-**
    industrial 122, *337*, **994-**
examination 123, *338*, **V70-**

Yawning, psychogenic 51, *71*, **3001**
Yaws 37, *31*, **136-**

Zona 32, *10*, **053-**
Zoster 32, *10*, **053-**